T0375509

MEETING THE
STRANGER WITHIN

Meeting the Stranger Within

Transformation of a Cancer Patient

Walter Hampton Baily

Copyright © 2007 by Walter Hampton Baily.

Library of Congress Control Number: 2007900466
ISBN: Hardcover   978-1-4257-5375-7
               Softcover   978-1-4257-5373-3

All rights reserved. No part of this book may be reproduced or transmitted
in any form or by any means, electronic or mechanical, including photocopying,
recording, or by any information storage and retrieval system,
without permission in writing from the copyright owner.

This book was printed in the United States of America.

To order additional copies of this book, contact:
Xlibris Corporation
1-888-795-4274
www.Xlibris.com
Orders@Xlibris.com
37167

CONTENTS

Also by the author, with Thelma Falk Baily:

CHILD WELFARE PRACTICE

A Guide to Providing Effective Services
For Children and Families

Jossey-Bass, 1983

DEDICATION

To all those who

By profession or

By personal commitment

Care for others.

Without you, we are all alone.

PREFACE

In January 2005, I decided to write about my experience with prostate cancer treatment and the variety of physical and emotional responses that I experienced. Each prostate cancer patient's treatment will vary, and each may experience different responses. It is my hope that this description of my own circumstances, responses, and recovery may help to provide a useful perspective for other prostate cancer patients, their family members, and friends.

Numerous sources of information were used for this book: descriptions of a variety of medications; my medical records from the three medical groups or physicians serving me; letters that I had sent to all three groups during the course of treatment; periodic notes that I kept during treatment; data from insurance records; observations of me by family, friends, and medical personnel; professional articles and research about prostate cancer from governmental and nongovernmental agencies; reports from cancer magazines, such as *Cure*; professional information from the Internet; my review of some books on cancer; and last, my recollection of experiences.

Three facilities in New England served me: one was a combined hospital and cancer center, the second was a major hospital, and the third was a community hospital. The names of all medical persons who attended me have been changed in order to protect their personal privacy.

ACKNOWLEDGMENTS

Appreciation is expressed for the many persons who encouraged me to write and who also read and critiqued materials. Everyone who read my material did so with dedication and generosity. Their observations not only enhanced the presentation; they increased my spirit to complete the effort.

Special thanks go to Janet Grieco, journalist, and now novelist and a board member of the Maine Writers and Publishers Alliance, who was gentle and clear about ways to improve the manuscript. The Xlibris staff and editors competently provided the final revisions to assure current language construction and attractive layout design.

Finally, thanks to all of the medical practitioners who worked together to bring about the successful treatment of my disease and who offered warm and humane care at all times.

CHAPTER 1

Walk into any waiting room in a prostate cancer treatment center, and sooner or later—more likely sooner—the following letters will be used—PSA. The conversation goes something like this:

"So what was your PSA when they referred you for treatment?"

"It was, uh, about 3.5 then moved up to a 4 in a short time, probably in about five months or so; then it jumped to 6.2. Didn't mean that much to me. My doctor said she wanted to take the test again, and if it didn't change, then she wanted me to see someone else."

"What was yours?"

"I was going along for a couple of years at almost 5, and then it jumped to 6.6, something like that, and they told me I had to get another exam since I may need some treatment for possible cancer. So I saw a urologist and then landed here for treatment."

A third man asks, "What about you?"

"My PSA was just creeping up slowly, then when it got to about seven, they said I better get this looked at. Right now, of course, it's almost zero. They told me that it would probably move up a little bit over time."

PSA stands for prostate-specific antigen. These initials become almost a part of one's identity. Once a man has prostate cancer, whether treated or not, this is a key indicator of the possible presence of cancer, as well as changes in the gland. The test is simple; a very small blood sample is taken, and the results are known in as little as two hours, if the lab gets the specimen quickly.

The general belief in the professional community is that every man should have a PSA test by age fifty. Others say age forty-five is better, and more recently the number by some specialists has dropped to forty, especially for men of African descent who have a higher rate of prostate cancer. If there is a family history, then men should start the PSA at least by age forty. Regardless of the recommendation that men get PSAs, one can read about physicians, even oncologists at age fifty and above, who have not yet had the test.

The prostate is a gland about the size and shape of a walnut that sits beneath the base of the penis and makes seminal fluid. The PSA test measures the level of a protein that is released into the blood by the prostate gland when it is irritated or inflamed. It is not a foolproof indicator of prostate cancer, but it is a rather strong guide to the presence of cancer. Conditions other than cancer may cause the PSA to rise. For example, a slight enlargement of the gland can cause a rise in the PSA score. Generally, a score under 4, even a bit more, indicates that cancer is unlikely. A score of 7 or more suggests the presence of cancer.

The PSA test, which has been around since about 1980, remains controversial. It is not clear at present whether a rising score is more or less important than the score itself. Some physicians claim that a number, such as 6 or 7, is a reliable indicator of the presence of cancer. Others say that the number itself means little; it is only the increase in the number and the speed (physicians use the word "velocity") of the increase that is important. Others say that for some men, neither way is reliable, and both numbers do little but cause alarm. Patients may go into treatment or worry extensively about cancer when they would do better to just ignore it or do some "watchful waiting." Testing can be continued until there are some very dramatic changes in the numbers. Then more extensive diagnostic procedures can be started.

In spite of sometimes-vociferous positions by medical researchers about the value of the PSA test, most physicians use it to monitor changes in the prostate gland. It is considered a useful test especially when combined with other diagnostic measurements. Researchers are currently examining other biological markers in the hope of finding a more precise blood-related diagnosis of prostate cancer.

My personal family physician, Dr. Maya Shah, had been following my PSA scores for almost three years. They were quite close and increasing very slowly until the last one jumped up rather quickly.

My numbers looked like this:

January 9, 2000   -   4.43
March 25, 2001   -   4.47
August 14, 2001   -   4.54
August 18, 2002   -   7.58

A week after the last one, Dr. Shah and I talked about the sharp increase in the score. She asked whether I understood what the higher number might mean.

"Well, I really don't except it suggests that I could be getting cancer on that gland. I know very few details other than that."

I had a minimum reaction to the question. I know that when I can't give a clear response or have concern about something, I may look away or give a small shake to my head in an I-don't-know gesture. I also know that if a person has to speak clearly in public on a subject with which he is not familiar, one can always mumble a few words until some thoughts can be pulled together. That's about what I did.

Dr. Shah said, "I wish we could have had another PSA sooner than this, since the number moved up a little. But we have to work from here." I agreed and told her that she had asked for another but that I had dragged my heels and didn't get one.

We talked about the possibility of cancer for a few minutes, and I listened carefully. She assured me that more study would have to be made to determine whether cancer was present, and if so, the extent of it. At the end, I simply shrugged my shoulders and said I would go ahead with what she recommended. She told me the best way to start is to see a urologist. These are specialists in the genitourinary system, and they both diagnose and participate in prostate cancer treatment. I agreed to see one, and she planned to call me when a time was set up.

An appointment was set for September 18, 2002, with a Dr. Tyson. Before the meeting, I talked to a friend who I knew had gone through prostate cancer treatment, and he had seen the same doctor. After hearing my friend's positive experience, I felt at ease about seeing Dr. Tyson. He was direct and clear, and he certainly seemed interested in helping me with this possible cancer. Our first meeting was a basic discussion of the first steps to obtain a diagnosis. I received several brochures on cancer, and on the way out, I picked up a few other folders to see what they said about cancer.

I read them a couple of times; and after finishing them, I had the well-here-we-go-again attitude, meaning I didn't know exactly what I was getting into, but I had to go through with it.

At the next meeting, Dr. Tyson performed a rectal exam. This is a quick and easy physical exam called the DRE or digital rectal examination. From now on, every time I see either an oncologist or a urologist, I will be given a DRE.

The physician places his or her index finger into the anus and the rectum area and feels about three-fourths of the surface of the gland with the last digit of the finger. This provides a quick assessment of the texture—the roughness or the smoothness—of the surface of the gland as well as the probable size and shape of the gland. One-fourth of the gland can almost never be reached because of the closeness of the bladder and the urethra, the tube that carries urine from the bladder and goes through the prostate. The exam takes about five seconds and gives a momentary feeling of fullness in the rectum. On my prostate, there was roughness on the surface of the gland; the roughness suggested the presence of cancer.

He then inquired about any abdominal pain. Did I have problems urinating, such as a slowness to start the flow, unusual pressure during urination, the need to frequently urinate, or never being able to empty the bladder at one time? I had none of these.

"Finally," he asked, "what about nighttime—do you have to get up often to urinate?"

"Just once a night" was my reply. He agreed that was about normal, in fact, pretty good for my age.

He asked these questions probably to determine whether I had BPH, benign prostatic hypertrophy, also called hypertrophic disease, which is an enlargement of the prostate gland. This expansion inhibits the free flow of urine through the prostate. Dr. Tyson said he felt no gland enlargement, but a later test would be more accurate. BPH affects about one in five men by age forty, one in two by age seventy-five, and 80 percent of men over age eighty. It is treatable.

"So what's next?" I asked. He told me there would be a bone scan, ultrasound and biopsy, and a full medical report from Dr. Shah. I got no more details, and I had learned by observation that patients moved in and out of his office rather quickly. Perhaps I could have asked more questions, but I asked none. At this point, I was more willing to get things underway for a diagnosis.

As I drove home that day, I began to think that time was eluding me and that I had not a moment to waste. I also began to feel that I was being hustled into treatment. Perhaps the cancer was worse than I thought, but no one actually told me that. But these appointments were quite close together, and I thought that must mean something—something bad. Now I wished that I had taken the PSA test earlier. Never a confirmed worrier, except about money, I was now starting to be one. I had more to worry about now than losing money. I could lose . . . well, yes, I could really lose; and just as I was thinking about that, I told myself I better pay attention to my driving.

A general physical exam is always needed to determine whether there has been any spread of cancer cells, especially to the lymph glands. A bone scan may also be needed to rule out the movement of cancer cells into other areas. Pelvic bones are close to the prostate, so these are the typical locations to which cancer cells will travel. I had a full body bone scan, and no spread had occurred.

Currently the most accurate indicators of prostate cancer include ultrasound and biopsy of the gland. Both of these tests may be conducted with the same instrument. A smooth probe, roughly the size of a very large thumb, is placed in the rectum and gently moved around by the doctor. First, the ultrasound unit is used to confirm the size and shape of the gland. All measurements are recorded on film. The urologist then moves the probe to the precise location of the gland to get samples. A one-inch needle emerges rapidly and extracts and retains samples from the gland.

Not all men need a biopsy. A PSA score of 7 or above is often used as the line beyond which a biopsy will be taken. Since my PSA was over 7.5, Dr. Tyson wanted to do biopsies on several parts of the gland to discover the extent and severity of probable cancer. I agreed to the test, knowing that it would be uncomfortable. The appointment was scheduled for November 1, 2002.

To say that this exam hurts is like saying that a lightning strike is a spark. The brochure I received on this procedure states that "this is slightly uncomfortable." I had read the entire brochure a couple of times and was prepared for some discomfort. First of all, I had known that I had a tight sphincter muscle, but this was not the problem. Dr. Tyson was gentle, and he used plenty of lubricant. But it was the biopsies that really hurt. Following each injection of the needle, which I could clearly feel, there was a sharp loud sound as if a small gun, like a .22-caliber rifle, had just gone off.

My worst fantasies emerge at times like this when I have no control over anything. I feel small and helpless. I began to worry more. When I heard the sharp noise, I was sure I had been shot. How quickly would he reload the gun? Then I knew this was not a diagnostic test; it was a new form of treatment. Tyson had found the gland, and he would not let it get away. He would kill it right now. My next concern was . . . and then I heard the shot again, and my fantasies stopped as quickly as they started. I had three biopsies, and each time I jumped slightly, although I was lying down. Dr. Tyson recognized that I was uncomfortable and asked, "Can you take one more that I'd like to get?"

At that point, I was breathing somewhat heavily; and as I caught my breath before saying anything, I responded very softly and as diplomatically as I could, "It would be very nice if you did not have to take another one."

He agreed and said that he did have three, and those would be a good indicator. He left the room, and as the nurse was cleaning up materials, I asked a question that I should not have asked. It was a stupid question. My voice was still soft.

"That was a tough exam; how did I do?"

Before she answered, I suddenly knew what the answer would be. After all, would she say that I was a total coward? No, her answer was simple, "Oh, you did fine with that."

A few months later, as three other men and I were in the cancer center awaiting treatment, I decided to ask them whether they had the biopsy and how they felt about it. All three had the exam.

The first man shook his head quickly and said, "It's the worst exam I ever had."

The second man nodded and said, "Yup, that's the way I feel too." He looked at the man next to him.

The third man was more crisp; his was a finality that closed off any further discussion: "I don't even want to talk about it."

That gave me some assurance that I was not too far off in my opinion.[1] A male physician wrote that part of the brochure, and I wondered whether he

---

[1.] In a later review of books by men who had the same biopsy, I found that I was not alone in my discomfort. Leon Prochnick, in *You Can't Make Love If You're Dead,* said that "having bits of sample tissue snipped from your prostate feels like having the inside of your behind attacked by a stapling gun." This was a large, muscular man who said that he felt like a wimp. Physicians are not immune from pain either. A pediatrician, F. Ralph Berberich, in *Hit Below the Belt,* said that "as the needle penetrated my rectum into the prostate, it stung a lot. In fact, it hurt like hell." This patient even had anesthesia. Another patient, Robert Fine, MD, was told that there would be a loud noise, and there was. Writing in *Prostate Cancer: A Doctor's Personal Triumph,* he stated that the "pin pricks were punches jammed deep inside me. The pain reverberated down through my balls. (The examining doctor) repeated the process five more times. I was exhausted when he finished, as much from the stress as from the pain."

had ever taken the exam.[2] The brochure also said that there would probably be some blood in both urine and feces for a few days afterward. I saw blood. It was a new experience, but at least I had been warned. It's what you have to do to get a diagnosis. All evidence of blood stopped after four days. While the bleeding was going on, I wondered if it would stop. After all, I was cut inside in several places. If you are cut on the inside, you can develop a serious infection. The brochure told me that. When I urinated, I saw blood—fresh blood—in the toilet bowl. *Bright red blood.* My blood. I didn't like it.

*   *   *

My son, Peter, who was home for a few days, drove me to Dr. Tyson's central office; and I was glad that he did. The three of us met after the exam, and Dr. Tyson explained that there were three lesions on the gland; by watching the ultrasound shadows and features, he suspected a fourth on the side he could not reach. It appeared that this was cancer, but he wanted to have this reviewed by other staff. I was given another appointment with him for the following week, November 6, 2002. He strongly recommended that a family member be with me to hear the observations. Peter and I talked about this as we walked to the car; he expressed concern for me. I knew he could not come back. I thanked him and said I would get a close friend to join me.

I told him how glad I was that he brought me there today. I didn't know how uncomfortable the exam would be. I then thought of Dr. Tyson's statement that, without any doubt, I had cancer. As we drove away, I looked at the grey sky. I felt the raw weather. Both reflected exactly the way I felt inside. Why does the weather have to be so miserable, so raw, when you

---

[2]   Following a Mayo Clinic study of two hundred and forty-three men who were given anesthesia prior to a biopsy, investigators noted that pain reduction is significant. They stated that patients should request anesthesia and that "pain control should be the standard of care in a urologist's office." *www.nim.nih. gov/medlineplus/news/HealthDay*, "Prostate Biopsy Doesn't Have To Be Painful," September 14, 2006.

feel so miserable inside? I didn't tell Peter how I really felt inside. Maybe he knew; in fact, I'm sure he knew.

This is a tough moment when you're a parent. In the natural sequence of life, the passage of time, parents are the ones who worry about their children. Children should not have to worry about their parents. It's just not the way life should be. I did not want him to worry about me, even though he is age fifty and very competent, very strong. For me, something is inherently wrong with that reversal, although I know it happens and will undoubtedly continue to happen as I get older. However, deep within my very being he will remain, in a very compressed form, the little boy my wife and I raised. I can perceive accurately the current man, but I can also see the entire arc of his life. No child, no matter how old and mature, should have to worry about the parent. That was the way I felt that day.

As we rode home together, I tried not to be despondent, but I was.

My other two children also lived in other states and could not be present for the next meeting with Tyson. I asked my friend, Denise, an RN who worked in the same medical group as my family doctor and in the same building as Tyson's local office to join me. She agreed to be there.

* * *

There was both rain and snow on the morning of the meeting, and I was very tired, having been up late the night before to watch returns on the midterm national elections. I don't follow politics intensely, but I become more absorbed at election time. I may have watched particularly late that night to distract me from what was coming the next day.

While I can have ideas and thoughts that can be described as humorous, or a few that may only be described as silly, I was beginning to have some bizarre ones, undoubtedly stimulated because my concerns about cancer became a larger proportion of my time. I was not aware at this early time in cancer diagnosis that stronger variations of such thinking would invade my mind. They would be induced primarily by the start of hormone therapy. Humor is clearly known to be therapeutic when persons face serious disease threats, and I found that mine helped to balance some of my distress. I don't believe that my behavior was ever erratic, but some of my thoughts certainly were.

Dr. Tyson's satellite office is in a one-story structure next to the hospital. It houses a half dozen physicians' suites. I arrived thirty minutes ahead of time, something I never do. This is not a welcoming waiting room; it is used by several visiting physicians on different days and also serves as a phlebotomy lab—one of those mysterious medical terms created by a sinister secret society in a dark dungeon that makes you wonder what ghastly torture will be inflicted when you walk in. To me the term is simply a weak attempt to conceal the fact that your blood will be extracted, and always more than you can spare.

This is not a place to put anyone at ease. Put simply, it is a dreary room. The chairs are old and packed together, and you hope the folding chair will not collapse when you sit down. The old metal coat hanger is usually full, so most people hold coats on their laps and look at their feet. Old magazines, usually of the kind that no one would willingly buy, let alone read, sit on weary tables. There are no windows. And why can I never find a man's magazine, such as *Popular Mechanics*, or maybe an automobile magazine? It is well known that the building will be torn down in a few years, and no one will be sorry.[3]

Conversations between some staff and patients are easily overheard in the hallway at this waiting room. You try not to listen, but there is no way to avoid hearing what is said. The entire building, some fifty years old, is for another age of medicine, not this one. A sign on the wall tells you to wash your hands often. Why bother? There are so many germs packed in this room that some days the patients can't get in.

Congestion is eternal in this tiny waiting room, caused by patients coming and going, including the constant trail of patients who are given a small clear plastic container by the receptionist, with a lid and a name or

---

[3.]   The entire building was demolished three years later.

a number on the top, and then directed to a very small bathroom. We all know exactly what they will do in there, since most people sitting in the room have done the same thing. Including me. So much for confidentiality and privacy. It's too bad that the hospital doesn't get creative and pipe in music, "Macarena", or conga, so the tight line of patients heading for the bathroom could kick and dance their way there and the rest of us could cheer them on. This would lighten up the whole place. Patients would beg to take a urine test. Those not getting the test would never look at their feet again. Patients would laugh, talk with glee about . . . . It'll never happen, but it's amusing to think about it.

*   *   *

The room was busy when I took a seat, the only one left. I did not expect to see Denise there, so I walked to her office down the hallway and left a message for her. I came back, but the seat was taken. I was getting edgy. I picked up an aged magazine, and the middle fell out of it. Then I remembered the hand-washing sign; I moaned to myself and put it down.

I looked again for Denise, wondering how soon she would arrive. I glanced over at Tyson's receptionist, wanting to ask her when I might be seen. She was unavailable at the back of an office. Should I go across the hall to find Denise? If I did, would I miss my time and have to wait still longer? Now my eyes were shifting back and forth, always hoping Denise would walk in. Five more minutes passed. I rose, walked quickly to her office once more, and left another message. I didn't care that this might annoy her; I needed her now. Right now. I did not want to see Tyson alone. I knew what he would say, but I did not want to hear it by myself.

To my relief, she walked in a few minutes later, cheerful and composed. I was neither. But I was grateful for her presence. I stood, we hugged each other, and she began to talk. There were a fewer people in the room when she arrived, but they were silent. Denise chatted about some inconsequential things. She continued to talk about things that did not interest me. I was surprised since she was so alert and sensitive to someone else's needs. I nevertheless listened and responded as best I could. That was a part of my training in social work graduate school. Keep yourself out of the discussion, only listen and respond to the other. It was one of the characteristics that enabled me to help others. This day I felt I had no strengths, no characteristics, no substance at all. I wanted to talk about myself a little bit, but I tried to respond to her.

My name was then called, and we walked to Dr. Tyson's examining room. Denise then asked how I was feeling, and I said almost abruptly I was really not concerned about myself.

"I know what Tyson is going to say—I have cancer, period." I said this firmly but also with resignation. I was short with her, which is not the way I act, especially with a friend like Denise. She tried again. I explained that I was far more concerned about my cousin who lived nearby and who was just diagnosed with a serious cardiac disease. Denise told me that she knew the doctor that my cousin would be seeing, and he would get good treatment. She gently suggested that I should think a bit about myself. Finally, I yielded to her request; and just as we started to talk a little about cancer, Dr. Tyson walked in.

He explained carefully the extent of my cancer. Several terms are used to describe the level of cancer. Mine was on the upper side of an intermediate risk cancer, with a Gleason score of 7 out of a total of 10. This score is derived from two sources: the stage of cancer development and the characteristics of the skin on the cancer nodules. Cancers were found on three parts of the gland, which gave a score of 4, and the cancer had not spread into the bone, so the stage was a 3. A Gleason score is also considered an indicator of the aggressiveness of the disease.

Treatment was recommended, and after a brief discussion, I was rather sure I did not want surgery. That sounded to me to be too radical a procedure. He accepted that but thought I should think about it a bit more and let him know later. He said that if I did not choose surgery, then he recommended that a first form of treatment would be a series of hormone injections to deprive the cancer of testosterone, which feeds the cancer. He recommended that it be started very soon so that further cancerous growth is inhibited. The medication is given either once a month or every three months, and it eliminates the majority of testosterone. I agreed to contact him within a week.

I heard the words "very soon." Very soon. That's what I was worrying about. They didn't tell me, and I didn't ask whether I was being rushed into treatment. But hormone treatment should start very soon. Was I too late in getting treatment? Would it go into the bones? That's where prostate cancer is serious. "Very soon." Words I would try to avoid, but not forget.

Denise and I walked back to her office together. I thanked her for staying with me. I started to talk generally about prostate cancer and treatment, saying nothing definite, just vague comments about how soon it can be over, how much it would be to go through treatment. I shrugged my shoulders in the noncommittal way I do. I felt a bit like a dog that has just come out of a pond and who immediately tries to shake all the water off. That's what I wished I could do. But I couldn't. All this talk, all this reading, and all this thinking about cancer were inside my head, inside me—just where the damned cancer was and was still growing, expanding. All this scary stuff was not on the surface of my skin. I couldn't shake it off. It was inside. I volunteered that surgery just seemed to me to be too drastic, although I had certainly read that men have it. I said that I just have to think about it, talk to my sons and daughter, and go from there. At that time, Denise had a patient waiting, and I was glad—quite glad—to try to forget everything and not talk about it.

The next day I glanced at a couple of the cancer brochures again and was reminded that surgery sometimes results in urinary incontinence. That information made me wince. My urinary system is not first class; it's an old model. Built in 1925, it has no flaws, requires no maintenance, and has never needed treatment. It's analog, not digital; there are no codes to punch in and no passwords.

To select surgery and possibly lose an important piece of equipment made me think more carefully. This is a bit like buying a house. Most people know that a house built before World War II is invariably of high-quality materials. It might be an old style, but more care was taken in construction—no substituting cheap replacements, no cutting corners. While there's no direct comparison between houses and a urinary system, that's the way I saw mine at the moment. It might be old, but it's still in good condition; best of all, it was constructed before World War II. Don't risk losing it.

Within a day or so, I read an article about men's diapers, and I winced once more. While in the supermarket to pick up paper goods, I saw adult diapers. I had never noticed them before. My body told me to withdraw from that space, back away, remove myself. This is not a safe place to stand. This is not something you want to see. Maybe when you're older, but not now. Certainly not now. I called Tyson and left a message: no surgery. NO. I was referred to the nearby cancer center for further treatment.

On December 11, 2002, I received my first injection of a medication to eliminate testosterone. This treatment is referred to as hormone therapy, and it is also referred to as androgen deprivation therapy. My PSA number dropped to 0.15 by March 5, 2003. At the end of July 2003, the number was 0.00. It has remained at zero for more than three years.

*   *   *

Prostate cancer is a lethal disease. It does kill, and it *may kill* unless treatment is obtained in time. Primarily a disease of older men, prostate cancer arrives with few warnings, often none. It is the original stealth disease. No symptoms. If there are symptoms, the cancer may have moved along with some speed. If it spreads, it often goes first to the pelvic bones. Then it's hard to treat. Bone pain is very difficult to manage. It can be an ugly death.

Prostate cancer strikes almost at the center of the male identity—at one's very manhood. Is that why men are reluctant to discuss it? What man wants to say in polite conversation that he has a disease "down there" or that he is impotent—or periodically impotent? Most men have little knowledge of the gland, either its location or its considerable role in the contribution to reproduction. Men know about their penis; some brag about size, shape, achievements, even conquests. With prostate cancer, that organ is now under threat, threat of impairment—possible termination of functioning with a partner. Is extinction too strong a word?

Erectile dysfunction, or ED, is the socially acceptable term today; and jokes are endless. But what man even wants to think that he may not be able to maintain an erection? That strikes real fear. The strong biological drive to have progeny, no matter the age, may be terminated. Two questions arise: "Is my life over?" "Can I love again?" Those questions possibly precede "Will I die?" How many reasons can men find to refuse any exam that is related to their sexual functioning or to life and death concerns?

The types of prostate cancer treatment may impair, short or long term, the management of urination, control of bowels, and sexual functioning. These are all areas for potential embarrassment and for reduced quality of life. They are also essential subjects for discussions with medical specialists.

The effects of prostate cancer are often, but not always, manageable and treatable if treatment is sought in time. Various national cancer groups state that about 232,000 men were diagnosed in 2005 with prostate cancer. For the year 2006, the number was increased to more than 234,000. The *Nutrition Action Health Letter* makes those numbers a bit more specific: "On an average day in the U.S., 640 men are diagnosed, while 75 die of prostate cancer."[4] Of those who are diagnosed with the disease, about half will receive radiation therapy. The bad news is twofold: blacks have a higher rate of prostate cancer than other groups; the disease kills slightly more than 30,000 men in a year. It is the third leading cause of death in males. The American Cancer Society gives the good news: the mortality rate for all men has very slowly begun to fall.

---

4.   *Men's Health*, "Checking Under the Hood," vol. 33, no. 6, July/August 2006, 2–7.

CHAPTER 2

"Your blood pressure is 155 over 83," the nurse said as she looked at the monitor. I had just taken off my outer coat and sat down at the cancer center and was still breathing a little heavily from moving fast through the hallways to get to this appointment on time.

"Well, that's a lot," I commented. "It's never that high; I think I know what's caused that." I smiled. "I had so much trouble parking outside; I thought I'd never find a place. And then the construction equipment seemed to be everywhere. I didn't want to be late for this first meeting. But finally I found a spot."

Suzanne, one of the nurses at the Radiation Oncology Division at the cancer center, had just introduced herself and gave me a friendly welcome. The date was February 26, 2003.

"It's true, parking is a problem here," she answered. "They keep telling us that the construction will finally end, but then the contractors keep extending the finish date. It'll be over in about three months, we all hope."

"My blood pressure is almost always in a normal range, something like 110 to 115 over 72 or 78," I suggested. I didn't want her to think I had high blood pressure.

"Does that automatic cuff always record pressure correctly?" I asked cautiously. "I've had them used on me a couple of times, and they were way off. So then when I was checked with the manual method, the pressure was much lower."

A manual cuff was not noticeable in this large area open to the hallway, and Suzanne didn't seem too concerned about it.

"Oh, it's all right," she said. "We always expect that when people show up here, their pressure is a bit high in the beginning."

"OK, that's good, but I do keep records on my blood pressure," I insisted. "Do you want me to bring in some recent numbers to you? I have the info at home."

"Oh no, that's not necessary, but thank you anyway."

As she was checking her file for a moment, Suzanne said, "Maybe you'll step on the scale over here, and we can check your weight."

"OK."

She adjusted the small weight on the rail. "It looks like one thirty-eight," she said, partly talking to herself as she recorded the information.

"One thirty-eight?" I inquired. "Gee, I'm usually not that high, but maybe it's my heavy shoes, or maybe . . . oh, well," I said quietly. Then, in a still lower voice but of sufficient volume so that Suzanne could hear me, I added, "I usually seem to be about 130 or so." She made no response but asked me to follow her to an examining room where she would request data for a medical history.

This appointment was for basic screening prior to receiving treatment for prostate cancer. Suzanne was obtaining basic medical data and checking on the accuracy of information already received. Soon I would meet Dr. Brooks, one of the oncologists in this service, who recently had sent me a letter asking me to come for pretreatment planning.

Suzanne asked about the typical items included in a history: hospitalizations, surgeries, allergies, family history of cancer, other cancers, use of tobacco and alcohol, significant weight changes, serious illnesses, cardiovascular problems, general health status, and current medications (only a baby aspirin).

My father died from a coronary infarction at sixty-seven; my mother died at eighty-four from congestive heart failure. I have no siblings. I smoked for about three years, starting in the navy in WWII and shortly afterward. Since that was so long ago, she was not sure whether to include that data.

Suzanne was more interested in the fact that I had about a dozen basal cell carcinomas removed and one squamous cell cancer removed from my hand. In addition, I had two much larger lipomas, commonly known as fatty tissues, removed from my shoulder blades (this was done under a local anesthetic, and I thought the growths looked like chicken fat). They were "mirror" growths, since they were in exactly the same position except on opposite sides of my back. Both were removed about two years apart; both were benign. I recently had some other skin problems, called topical dermatitis and not related to cancer; and they were treated by some prescription lotions.

Dr. Harold Brooks then came in, introduced himself, and welcomed me to the center. He was relaxed as he asked me many questions and gave me information about the services there. I felt so comfortable that I thought I was a guest at a spa. But much later, with the power of the radiation treatment I was to receive, I would not feel so comfortable.

We reviewed some of the same medical information I had given to Suzanne. He asked about any heart problems, since he noticed that the only pills I took were the daily 83 mg of aspirin.

I told him that I had two admissions presumably for heart symptoms. Neither case turned out to be a heart attack; and the first event, five years ago, was caused by my own activities one afternoon. I worked in the kitchen in winter next to a wood stove—obviously in very dry heat—with a skill saw and inhaling wood dust then ate very little supper, had a cup of coffee and a very rich piece of cake, and finally varnished a kitchen worktable I was making for my daughter. I did that in a closed room. My only excuse was that I would dash out of the room, inhale fresh air, and go back in. I knew it was ill advised, but I was absolutely determined to get it finished. The table almost finished me off. It turned out to be a great table. By midnight, I was in the ER.

The second event occurred several years later, when I had almost all the symptoms of a cardiac problem. Four days later, I was discharged and the physician told me my heart was fine, and he called me an anomaly. A physician friend told me, "You had the best kind of heart attack." I told Dr. Brooks that I just may be lucky.

"Any follow-up with a cardiologist?"

"Yeah, a number of times, but my heart has always been normal."

"Any cancer in the family?"

"An uncle died of throat cancer at ninety-two, and an aunt died at age seventy-five—both of them were on my mother's side."

"Any other serious illnesses in the family?

"No, not really."

"So you seem to be in fairly good health now; is that pretty accurate?"

"Well, I think so, yes." I nodded my head in agreement.

"How physically active are you?"

"Well, depends on the time of year. In the dead of winter, not very, but I take care of a good-sized woodlot, cutting limbs off trees, cutting firewood, keeping roadways and trails open, all of which I like to do, so that means I am quite active in the better weather."

He then asked, "Are you still having erections?

I paused for a moment and said, "They had slowed down a few years back and then essentially stopped about two years ago." He asked no more about this, although I thought he would pursue it further.

He then wanted to know more about me, what hobbies I have, my past work experiences, and the like. In my mind, I gave him very high marks for starting this way. This beginning allowed me and any other patient the opportunity of describing some of our work and interests, rather than being seen only or primarily as a disease attached to a person. I had absolute confidence that this was a genuine question and not just an automatic part of the intake discussion. I felt quite at ease in talking with him.

I quickly listed my work as a social worker in two mental health services—in a children's hospital in Philadelphia and in the public health arena. Following doctoral work in social research, my wife and I served as professors at the undergraduate level. About twenty-five years ago, my wife, who had worked extensively in children's services, and I started to work together as child welfare consultants and traveled frequently for our work. Together we wrote practice manuals and policies in child protection and helped states develop definitions of abuse and neglect. That work came to a conclusion with her death in 1996. I considered more work, but my children suggested I focus my energies on other interests, and I did. I realized I had worked until age seventy, and now my work on my woodlot and related environmental issues gives me considerable pleasure. I added that I liked health work and always felt comfortable in hospital or medical settings.

I was glad that we met in a well-lighted examining room with large windows and without the clutter of a desk and phone calls. If he had a cell phone, it was not evident, and there were no interruptions during this half-hour conversation. I felt that this entire reception reflected the respect that he, and probably this entire service, held for patients.

"Well," he said, "let's talk about your treatment here. What do you understand about your cancer?"

Prior to this question, Dr. Brooks and I were sitting about five or six feet from each other. But with that comment, he moved his chair much closer to mine, and the focus was entirely on my cancer and on treatment.

"Well, I guess it is just the basics," I said. "Dr. Tyson, the urologist who has seen me several times, explained that the prostate gland has three lesions or growths on it; and there is probably a fourth."

I explained that he could not absolutely determine the presence of the fourth because of its location, but I believed it appeared to be there from some shape or shadow on the ultrasound part of the test. My PSA test had jumped up quickly, and that test apparently is a fairly good proof of cancer. I also explained that when Dr. Tyson gave me the digital exam, he could feel the presence of roughness on the surface of the gland, and that again suggested some cancerous growth.

"I think that is what I understand also," Dr. Brooks said then asked, "How did you come to choose this center for your treatment?"

"Well, in a sense I may not have necessarily chosen it," I replied, "but I was referred by Dr. Tyson. It seemed best to come here."

I told him that I thought that I had better come here, based on getting treatment the soonest. We talked in our family about this disease, and it was my understanding from the urologist that it was starting to move along at an increasing speed. I thought it was best to stay with Tyson rather than seeking someone else since that would be starting all over and would only delay treatment. The other two choices probably were a good distance away, and one of them was in another state.

I then shifted the subject slightly and said, "Tyson had given me some literature from his office, and I understand that seed implants are often used successfully to treat this type of cancer. A friend of mine, a couple of years older than I am, had the implants done and said it was very easy—only a few hours of surgery, and that was it."

He nodded, and I asked, "Will I be able to get the implants here?"

"Well, no, we've looked at all your material and believe you need something stronger than that for the level of your cancer. Seeds are good when there is more time to treat it, but you will need a slightly stronger form of treatment, and that is radiation."

"Oh," I responded. "So that will mean I have to come here periodically or maybe fairly often?" I am sure there was dismay in my voice.

"Right. Currently we believe that you should receive about eight to nine weeks of radiation. That would be five days a week."

"Oh, that's quite steady, five days a week! Well, I didn't expect anything like that—quite a difference from seed implants." I could almost feel my insides drop down a bit. This was not what I wanted to hear. This would cut into all the things I wanted to do this spring in my woodlot and garden.

"Yes, it really is," he said with a look of understanding that I might not like this. He said something else here, but my mind was still back trying to comprehend the eight-week statement, and then I heard, "We have found that the consistency of the radiation is the important factor in containing the cancer and destroying it. X-ray is not nearly as effective if it is spread out over a longer time." I could not take it all in as quickly as he said it. My face probably looked like a white plaster mask with eyes fixed in a locked position.

He explained that the intensity and frequency of the radiation is what creates the cure. That's the reason it's important to be treated every day and not to miss any time unless there is a really good reason to miss time.

"Every day, huh? All right, well, I guess I can do that. I was planning on visiting my son in Boston in a few weeks, but just for a couple of days." I was groping for some way to avoid eight to nine weeks.

"Well, sometimes patients do have to take a day or two off," he said. "We understand that, but the best thing you can do is to be here every day during that time. Have you heard much about radiation for prostate cancer?"

"No, not really. Does it tire you out as treatment does for women who have breast cancer?" I asked.

"It will vary from person to person, but the simple answer is yes."

He explained that many women who receive chemotherapy find it very, even extremely, tiring. I would be most tired toward the end of the treatment period. Radiation is not only effective in killing the cancers, but it also destroys normal cells in the abdomen. Most men have trouble with their bladder and bowels. But there are medications to reduce pain or discomfort when that happens. Because radiation kills normal cells, it is essential that no radiation be given on weekends. It is coincidental that treatment is effective in five-day units. The body needs two days to recover from the negative effects of the radiation. The radiation equipment now in use is very precise in focusing exactly on the cancerous parts of the gland. The scatter around the primary beam is absolutely minimal, but at this stage of beam development, some scatter of the rays does occur.

"Dr. Tyson told you, I suppose, that the Lupron Depot[5] hormone medication you are taking is a way of controlling the cancers?" he asked.

---

5. Lupron Depot is one of a number of testosterone-suppressing medications. It is usually referred to in this book by its shortened name, Lupron. It is also described as hormone therapy. The term "androgen deprivation therapy" is frequently used in scientific reports.

"Yeah, he mentioned that; I gather that the Lupron stops the production of testosterone, and that deprives the cancers of nourishment, if that's the right word."

"Correct, and you've had a first injection?"

"Yes, that was on, mmm, let me see, December, the eighth, I think," I said. "It was a one-month quantity, but they also have a three-month dose. For the moment, I'm thinking that I would prefer the single month, since the other seems to me to be a large amount to get. That is a large amount of medication to have in your body at one time, even though it is time released. I guess the good part of the three-month dose is that I would only have to see the doctor every third month . . . saves a trip or two."

"Right. Many men choose the three-month injection for that very reason. You do have another appointment set up with Tyson?"

"Yes, in just about a month," I answered.

"Well, let's talk a little about the radiation procedure. First we put small tattoos on your abdomen . . ."

"Tattoos—really?" I smiled. "How big?"

"Tiny, here's one right here." He put his wrist in front of me, and there was a very small dark blue dot on the underside of his right wrist.

"Oh, that is small."

"You'll have three of them," he said. "One in the very center of your abdomen, very close to your penis, and one on either side of the abdomen and very close to the hip bone. These are used to establish the exact place where the radiation beam will be aimed."

He added that five beams of radiation would be given each day, one directed at each dot and two directed at midpoints between the middle one and the lower ones. I would be placed on a table under the radiation unit. It would move quietly over my body then stop to determine the exact place to send the X-ray. The radiation contains the precise amount and extent of power needed to destroy the cancer. The whole process would only take a few minutes. Two radiation therapists would be there each day to help set me up.

"I think you'll discover it is a rather simple process, not complicated at all," he said. "So how does this sound? Any questions or concerns about any of this?"

"No, I don't think so; it all seems quite clear. I have to admit I was not expecting this kind of plan. I really did have my mind set on the uhh . . . seed implants. Oh, well, it's obvious from what you say that I need the longer treatment. It did seem to me that I was being hustled pretty quickly into treatment, so I appreciate how quickly you have taken me into this program." No matter how cooperative or accepting I seemed to be, I was still wrestling with this high-powered schedule and what I knew was a long trip every day. Five days a week. Five days a week. I wanted to say, "No thanks."

"Good. Well, you'll probably have some questions as we go along, and I'll be seeing you every week throughout the time you are here to help with any concerns you have. And other staff will help you as needed. And now, how about you moving over to the table here and let me do a quick digital exam." He was referring to the digital rectal exam whereby the index finger is placed in the rectum and the surface of the prostate gland can be felt.

"Oh, sure, but let me use the bathroom first, since I find that it's best to have an empty bladder and bowel with that exam; it reduces the pressure on that area." I didn't want to have any embarrassing loss of control during the exam.

Dr. Brooks agreed and, after the quick exam, said that the gland felt the same as what was described in a recent report. He then explained that a staff member would place the tattoos on my abdomen. Next week there would be a short orientation by several staff to acquaint me with essentially all aspects of treatment, set up the time for the daily radiation X-rays, take some provisional X-rays of my abdomen, and program the machine for my particular treatment needs.

Dr. Brooks, in summing up our conversation, said, "It's rather clear from current records and current tests that you are in rather good health, and that definitely helps a person who goes through radiation, which is fairly strenuous on the body. The idea is, the healthier you go in, the healthier you come out."

"Thanks," I said, "that's very nice to hear. I did wonder about a person of my age getting treatment. After all, I am a bit older."

I told him that I could see that this will be quite costly although I have two insurances, and now I've just learned it will take a long time. Furthermore, at this age I don't know how much longer I will live. So that's something that I suppose a treatment center has to think about.

"Well," he added, "if you look at it from a purely statistical perspective, since you've reached this age without a really serious disability or chronic disease, you've got the likelihood of living another ten years. And, depending on any other events, you could live still longer than that." He smiled at me, probably because of the look of surprise on my face.

I didn't have a quick response to that but to thank him and say, "I have to admit that I have been very fortunate with my health."

Following the discussion with the doctor, I met with Andrea, one of the radiology therapists to have the tattoos placed; it was a simple procedure. I felt some mild movements on the skin surface. We talked briefly; I thanked her and left for the day. I learned later that Andrea would be one of the therapists meeting me in the treatment room. She and several of her colleagues would be more than professional in helping me through what would become an arduous treatment experience. Therapists are the key, first line staff who meet and assist patients every day.

*   *   *

The type of radiation that I would receive is called external beam, in contrast to internal beam. It is also referred to as XRT, meaning external beam radiotherapy. External therapy provides highly focused radiation to the gland. Mine would be 3-D conformal radiation beamed from five locations toward the gland. I had also started antiandrogen therapy, often called hormone therapy. This blocks almost all of the production of the testosterone hormone.

Internal radiation, which is what I had hoped to receive, is the insertion into the abdomen, or the prostate gland itself, a number of radioactive seeds about the size of rice grains. The seeds remain radioactive for about a year and are not removed from the body. Seed implantation, under anesthesia, takes about two hours. Obviously, this procedure is notably different from what I would receive.

Radiation side effects are considerable; the number and strength of these depend partially upon the strength of the radiation beams and the number of treatment days required. One federal government booklet[6] states that patients become very tired as treatment continues. "Patients may have diarrhea or frequent and uncomfortable urination." It can cause hair loss in the pelvic area, and skin in the "treated area may become red, dry and tender." Hair loss may be temporary or permanent. Some men may become impotent.

A National Cancer Institute booklet[7] refers to acute and chronic side effects, with the latter showing up some years later. Low energy and tiredness are common effects, including feelings of weakness. Dietary changes are recommended to maintain nutrition and body weight. It is not uncommon to lose one or two pounds a week during radiation. "Nearly all patients being treated for cancer report feeling emotionally upset at different times during therapy. It's not unusual to feel anxious, depressed, afraid, angry, frustrated, alone or helpless." Bowel problems, including pain and bleeding, are not mentioned in either pamphlet; but the cancer center staff was well aware of them.

The effects from all forms of hormone therapy are well established, depending upon the type of hormone received and the length of treatment. In a clinical review section of the *Journal of the American Medical Association* in July 2005, the side effects were listed as "decreased libido, impotence, hot

---

6.   *What You Need to Know about Prostate Cancer,* Public Health Service, U.S. Department of Health and Human Services, Washington, D.C., 1996, 18.

7.   *Radiation Therapy and You,* National Institutes of Health, National Cancer Institute, U.S. Department of Health and Human Services, Washington, D.C., 2001, 27–40.

flashes, osteopenia (mild bone loss, a precursor to osteoporosis), metabolic alterations and changes in cognition and mood."[8]

The American Association of Retired Persons (AARP) has a health telephone service, and it lists more events that might occur.[9] While a few overlap with the above items, several are a little more worrisome: impotence, nausea, peripheral swelling (in the limbs), transient bone pain (especially during the first week of therapy), vomiting, increased probability of osteoporosis, tiredness and low energy, delayed toxicity, enlargement of male breast tissue, and last, testicular atrophy, i.e., a wasting away of tissue, possibly from reduced sexual activity.

*   *   *

Within the first two minutes of my first contact, one can see by my responses the possible seeds of problems that could emerge during my treatment at the center. While I might need treatment, I was in effect saying that I knew my body fairly well and might perceive it more accurately than the center does.

By questioning the accuracy of their equipment and measurements, I was also saying that I might resist being dependent on them.

What also emerged here was a brief preoccupation with a very minor concern, namely, my weight. That would show up later in a somewhat amusing way.

With these three factors rather neatly buried within me, I would nevertheless become a cooperative patient, albeit weary, resistant, and weeping a number of times along the way. I may have created more problems for myself than I *otherwise* would have experienced. But I couldn't do much

---

8.   Nima Sharifi, MD, et al. "Androgen Deprivation Therapy for Prostate Cancer," *JAMA*, Journal of the American Medical Association, vol. 294, no. 2, July 13, 2005.

9.   AARP Nurse Healthline: American Association of Retired Persons, Health Information and Education, 1-888-543-5630.

about them at the time, since I believe I was unable to consciously recognize them.

I did not know how fortunate I was. My oncologist, Dr. Brooks; my personal physician, Dr. Shah; my family; the radiation therapists; and other cancer center staff did help me change my behavior as a patient, even though it took quite awhile.

After this meeting, it was clear that I would be taking a trip that I would not anticipate. I had to travel through seven towns, stop at seven traffic lights and ten stop signs, and travel forty-three miles each way five days a week for eight and a half weeks. The bad news—it was a long daily trip. The good news—spring was approaching; I might not face any severe snowy weather. As it turned out, the bad weather was on the weekends. I was never late and never missed a day of treatment.

CHAPTER 3

The room into which I walked each day for radiation is on one end of the building, with one side against the outside wall. Two other sides face interior rooms of the oncology center, such as a small waiting room, nursing station, and others. On the other side, adjacent to the entrance, is a control room with phones, computer screens, and a keyboard where oncology therapists monitor equipment functioning during the administration of the radiation. Entrance to the treatment room is through a double door and then down a gentle grade for twenty feet, then left into an open area that has a fairly high ceiling.

The room is essentially square, about thirty-five feet each way. In the middle is what can best be called a high-tech table, the top of which has a clear, hard plastic surface on which patients lie down to receive the radiation beams or units. Looking through from the top, one can see part of the structure of the table and other complex-looking parts. The table is just wide enough to hold a person comfortably and narrow enough for the staff to adjust a person to a precise location on the table. There are cabinets to the right as one enters; and strong linen/cotton cloths are stored there for use, two of them, by each patient on each visit. A few bright lights recessed in the ceiling seem to struggle to light one side of the room, since all the walls and ceiling are almost black, or at least so dark in color that it is difficult to define a color.

Hovering slightly above the table and set against the opposite wall from the entrance at the bottom of the ramp is the large bulbous radiation unit.

Officially known as a linear accelerator, it would be easy to ascribe animate features to this somber device with its large rounded surfaces and call it a very dark animal with smooth fur. The long arm that reaches out and above the patient is quite thick with an enlarged end that rotates around the patient. Powerful radiation beams are emitted from the end of the unit; they destroy cancer cells but also weaken or kill some healthy cells. In addition to the daily radiation units, the machine also performs regular and specialized X-rays once a week. These are used to determine any change in the size, shape, and location of the prostate gland; and when there are changes, a physicist recalibrates the focus of the beam.

In spite of the size of this equipment, the accelerator seems to have its own delicacy by the way it smoothly and effortlessly moves along and around your body. The prescription for my treatment included five stops for sending radiation beams: one directly above the abdomen, one from each side, and two at forty-five-degree angles on each side. Considering the therapeutic power of this machine, it is easy to ascribe both sophistication and intelligence to it, far beyond its physical composure. Consider this: not one of the human senses can assess the strength or even the presence of the health-giving energy emerging from the head of the machine. No one is able to taste, touch, smell, see, or hear anything when it performs its healing functions. The very name of the type of X-ray beam used—intensity-modulated radiation therapy—suggests, or perhaps even demands, that it should be accorded deference and respect.

There are no lights in the ceiling directly above the radiation unit. Because of limited lighting above it, it leaves a little more to the imagination of its exact shape or precisely how it functions. The room never seems bright, even when the lights are on. When the staff leave the room before the radiation beams begin their work, the overhead lights are turned off, and a small night-light remains on. While there are outlines of objects in the room, there is very little to see. Depending on the amount of light available, the accelerator appears to be a mix between light brown and a soft gray. Yet when I have looked at it as it hovered over my body, and as my eyes adjusted to the darkness, it turned to a soft tan color. I found the color rather soothing whenever I lay on the table.

What may be most notable upon entering the treatment room are the two fine red laser beams shining from two sides of the room. They intersect at the precise middle of the room, about three feet from the floor and at the midpoint of the table. These lights are the guides for the staff to place the patient in a prescribed location on the table.

When I entered the treatment room, I was met by one of the two therapists. One of them held a strong white cotton sheet in front of me at the beltline. This afforded personal privacy as I let my trousers and undershorts drop. I would then lie down on my back on a second white sheet in a certain location on the table. Staff members, standing on either side of the table, then moved me from side to side and back and forth, using only the sheet, until I was aligned with the beams. I was placed in a perfectly parallel line with the side of the table. A mild restraint was placed on my ankles to keep them upright and together and to minimize any possible leg movement.

I was located on the table so that the lowest, central tattoo mark on my abdomen, the mark directly above the shaft of the penis, was aligned exactly with the laser beams. A second purpose of the sheet placed in front of me was to prevent the penis from falling back on the abdomen or resting over the tattoo mark. If this should happen, then the penis would be fully exposed to the radiation beam, thereby contributing to genital discomfort. My position on the table was essential for the beams to precisely strike the cancerous lesions on the prostate gland, and nothing else. One of the two therapists adjusted the table surface up or down to reach the exact height of the intersecting laser beams. When properly positioned, one of the red beams shined on, or was directly over, the center of my nose. When the therapists left the room and the double doors were closed, it was quiet.

This is not a Frankenstein setting with blinding bolts of lightning, crashes of thunder, bubbling beaker jars, crackling electrodes, and crazed scientists in white jackets hysterically celebrating. Unless a person is uncomfortable about a large object, somewhat ominous in size moving closely over and around the head and body, it is calm. It is tranquil. It is restful. The only sound in the room is your own shallow breathing and the soft hum of the linear accelerator.[10]

Face the truth: this could be the best part of your day. You are lying down; you can close your eyes; the phone will not ring; the radio will not announce another crisis; you will not be pressured to buy something; you do not have to take out the garbage; you are not caught in a traffic jam; and you will feel no discomfort. You are instructed to be still, to breathe gently, and not to move.

With the very soft kittenlike purr of this ingenious man-made creature, you can contemplate peacefully and gratefully the daily destruction of your cancer cells. Or, at last, you can meditate, say a prayer, or be thankful that for once you are alone and isolated from this busy, frantic world. This respite from reality does not last long, maybe four, perhaps five minutes, depending on the amount of exposure required for your particular need.

Then it's up and out. "Thanks, see you tomorrow."

I wish that all medical therapies could be so easy.

---

[10]. Two years after my radiation treatment was completed, I learned that this room was specifically and carefully designed to provide a relaxed and comfortable environment for the patient. In my judgment, the designers succeeded admirably.

CHAPTER 4

On Thursday, March 13, 2003, the fourth day of radiation treatment, I woke up a bit early since my son, Peter, was leaving to go home and back to his employment. I was tired since I had awakened twice from the hot flashes and had to get up and use the bathroom. I also had a bad dream—in fact, a very upsetting one. I was sluggish and more or less had to drag myself out of bed. Peter and I had breakfast together, and I then helped him to pack and leave for home. I thanked him for being with me for a number of days and for driving me for the orientation meetings, various radiation measurements, and the first couple of days of treatment at the cancer center.

After showering, I still didn't feel much better and wished I did not have to go to the cancer center; but I was determined not to miss a single day, especially at the very beginning of radiation treatment. The weather was overcast and chilly, and I was anticipating spring weather. I always look forward to those days when there is bright sun on the snow that creates additional light.

Better yet is the cool breeze that comes across the top of the snow and the opposing warmth from the direct rays of the springtime sun. This balance of increased sun heat and cool air from the departing snow is, for me, the guarantee that spring is very close; and winter will soon be gone. But that was not today's weather. Nevertheless, I was glad that no snow was falling.

I arrived on time for the fourth radiation session. After walking in the back door, I stopped at the small refreshment table near the entrance and picked up some coffee and a muffin. I was about to go into the men's waiting room when I noticed a couple of other men in there. Since I was so weary, I did not wish to talk with anyone today. I chose to stand about thirty feet from the radiation room entrance where one of the staff could see that I had arrived. I knew I was apprehensive, edgy, even agitated; and I didn't know why except for being very tired and in what I would usually call a foul mood.

As I waited, I ate the small muffin quickly and then sipped the coffee in tiny amounts. It did not taste good to me this day, although the center provided a good quality of coffee.

Andrea and Howard were the two therapists who would be greeting and adjusting me on the table beneath the radiation unit today. I had just met them three days ago and was impressed with their gentleness, competence, and skill in relating to a patient. I thought they comprised a perfect team. Andrea came out to greet me, and we had just passed through the doors into the radiation room when she asked, "And how are you today?"

"Oh," I replied, "ahh . . . uuh, think I'm feeling a bit down."

And a split second after that, I felt my eyes filling with tears, and I began to cry. I simply did not know what was happening to me. As soon as she asked, I said to myself, "I wish no one had asked me that question." I believed that if I had not been asked, then I might not have started to cry.

By this time, we had walked down the ramp and had stepped into the radiation room where Howard was waiting for us. He already had a large white cotton sheet in his hands, ready to place it in front of me as I dropped my trousers to sit and then lie down on the table. But I was now fully crying, tears down my face, and I couldn't slow myself down.

Both of them made reassuring comments, saying that it was all right to weep and that other men have had upsetting experiences when being treated by radiation.

"Oh, uhhh . . . well, thank you." I paused for a moment. "I just don't know what is the matter with me today, but I feel terrible." Then I mumbled something about embarrassment. Again, their comments were gentle, stating that they had seen this many times; and it's OK here. But I was very ashamed of what had happened; I was equally baffled about my sudden tears.

Andrea said, "Are you OK to have the radiation now? Do you want to wait a bit, and we can do it a little later?" Howard confirmed what she asked.

"Nooo," I said softly, as I took a tissue from my pocket, paused as if I did not know what I was doing, then wiped my eyes. "Ahh . . . thanks, but, yeah, this will be OK now."

I lay down on the table. They adjusted me into the correct position for the radiation and made some comforting statements to me. I was still softly crying and didn't know why. Before they left, both of them checked with me again, saying, "Walter, are you all set?"

"Yes . . . I think I'm OK, thank you." My response was not very spirited. I was afraid to say much for fear that I would hear my pathetic voice, and I would just start crying more than I already was.

As I lay on the table, I remembered how important it was to remain in a fixed position with my arms at my sides. I continued to cry softly; and now as the tears emerged from my eyes, they came down the side of my face, partly into my ears and dropped on the table. It was a strange sensation. By the end of the radiation, I was not openly crying. But I still felt so dismal, unhappy to the point of asking myself, "What the hell is wrong with me? What is the matter with me?" I sighed a number of times to myself, as if this breathing would help me to know why I was crying.

Andrea came in first and asked how I was, and I made a rather general statement that I was feeling a little better, but I really wasn't. In her straightforward and clear manner, she said softly, "Dr. Brooks would like to see you now; can you stay awhile to meet with him? You probably remember that he wants to meet with you once a week?"

"Oh yes, I do recall that. Thanks for letting me know, and yes, I can stay awhile to meet him."

Howard added, "If you walk over to the nursing station, Suzanne, one of the nurses, will be there." I nodded in agreement.

"Thanks, I'll see you tomorrow," I said.

*   *   *

I immediately wondered to myself whether it was coincidental that my weekly meeting with Dr. Brooks happened to be on this day or was it quickly organized because of my upset. If the latter, I could quickly see that they were well organized and that their response was immediate when a patient is in apparent distress.

I dreaded the thought of walking the short distance to the station with some tears on my face; but I did that and, in fact, had no choice about it. I was ashamed to have what I knew must be a reddish face, moisture around my eyes, all perfect evidence that I was crying. Suzanne immediately greeted me.

"Hi, Walter, let's go over to this room here; and Dr. Brooks will be in shortly." Suzanne had my chart in her hand but was more interested in knowing how I was.

"How are you, Walter, what's happening?" she asked.

"I don't know what is the matter with me today." And then I began to cry more noticeably again. "But I do know I am very lonely, feeling very isolated from everything."

I told her how I suddenly missed my wife immensely and was very sad about that. I was very sad thinking about her just before I arrived. She died almost seven years ago—her birthday would be at the end of this month. I repeated that I did not understand what was happening to me. I began to repeat myself, saying again that I just did not know why I was so upset. I added, "I'm embarrassed; I don't . . . ahhh, I just don't act this way."

She offered me several tissues, and I continued to weep more quietly. My head was down. Suzanne was patient and let me talk and calm down a bit. I started talking aimlessly and explained, "We had been very happy together, worked together on various child welfare contracts for nineteen years, and she died while I was out of town. No way to say goodbye—no way." I paused for a moment. "It might be strange to say, but I still miss her . . . simply miss her."

I went on to describe how I had tried not to blame myself for her death, but it is hard to erase some events. I left to visit our daughter in Michigan when my wife was not feeling well, but she assured me she was all right. Two days later she died at home, but at least my son and daughter-in-law were with her. She absolutely refused to go to the hospital. She was a very private person about her health, and that characteristic was both her strength and then our loss.

With my head still facing down, I told how she was wary of doctors, and for some good reasons. She was once hospitalized and pulled every trick in the book to get out. But once, she had no choice about going to the hospital. I just picked her up, put her in the car, and took her to the emergency room. That was that: no argument.

As I slowly described these few facts about my wife, I became more calm, but I still had tears on my face. I continued to look down at the floor.

"Well, this is a real compliment to the good marriage that you and your wife had, and it's also a tribute to the joy and strength of your marriage."

I thanked her for listening.

"How soon do you think you'll be leaving?"

"Well, I'm not sure yet, guess I'll have to think about lunch," I said.

"What I'd like to know is whether you can get home safely by yourself," she asked.

"Oh, oh . . . aahh . . . I see. Yes, yeah, I can get home OK; Uh . . . I'm sure I can. I'll be fine, thanks." My voice was drab, flat, with a very depressed tone.

Just about this time, Dr. Brooks arrived. As Suzanne left, I thanked her for sitting with me.

Dr. Brooks and I said hello; he asked how I was. I told him in essence about my wife, how I suddenly felt very lonely and sad. I cried a little bit, but not in the same way as before. I was simply sad. My face was probably reddened, and he offered me a couple of tissues.

"Do you think you have any illness coming on, anything special that's bothering you?" he asked.

"No, I don't think so; it all just happened this morning," I replied. "I didn't sleep very well; in fact, I got very little sleep, and then I had a very bad dream, very upsetting. I was very restless; it was really a nightmare," I said.

I told him that when I got to the center, I was just miserable. Then when Andrea asked me how I was, I just could not hold myself together, just started to cry.

He waited for me to say more.

"The one small thing I do know is that I heard something on the radio coming down, probably a piece of music that reminded me of her, that is, my wife; and I got very sad . . . uhh . . . lonely.

"When you think about this even now, do you think there is anything that we could have done to prevent this sudden upset?"

"Well, I'm not sure, I don't think I'm sure about anything right now," I responded. "But, let me give it a thought, I just don't know."

"Yes, please think about that."

Dr. Brooks asked a few questions related to how I was doing otherwise, any abdominal problems, any upsets from food, problems urinating, any bodily changes that I was aware of.

"Well, the hot flashes are a pain, and they waken me at night—constantly—but they had started a while ago, and I guess they aren't much different from before," I replied. "They're very aggravating at times, and they were something I knew would happen. Urinating seems to be all right"

He waited for a few minutes as I became more settled. I had nothing else to say except, "I apologize for what's happening here, and . . . uhh, well, that's about it."

He wished me well, added that he would be here and would talk to me if I wanted to see him before I left today. I nodded, and my eyes avoided his. We agreed to meet again next Thursday. I sat alone in the room for several minutes to try to get myself composed and to rinse my face. When I left the room, I walked to an exit where the least number of people could see me.

I would later learn, in thinking about the several days preceding this event, and especially the frightening dream from the night before, that many factors had combined to cause this upset. In retrospect, it is surprising that I was not more upset.

CHAPTER 5

D_r. Brooks and I met again on March 27, 2003, two weeks after my upset. We greeted each other in one of the examining rooms. He asked about me, and I described no special changes. I then said, "I have thought about what happened two weeks ago; in fact, I may have found the source or the sources of the problem, or at least a significant part of it."

I mentioned several of the events that just preceded my weeping and that I had jotted a few things down. He seemed interested in hearing this and asked if I would be willing to write it down. I agreed.

When we met the following week, I told him that I had a letter almost completed and would get this to him shortly. He inquired how I was doing since last week, and I explained there were no basic changes. I felt a bit of abdominal discomfort, but not that much. I continued to be tired, much of it related to lack of sleep. Hot flashes awakened me three times a night consistently. I told him I was still hanging in there.

He said, "I've been thinking about you this last week and realize that you're spending a lot of time each day on cancer treatment. I know that it takes you almost an hour and a half by the time you get here, use the bathroom, sit down a minute or so, have some refreshment, and then go for the radiation."

He pointed out that it then takes the same time to get home. He knew that I ate at the hospital cafeteria occasionally, since we had seen each other there. He knew that I was not employed, although I worked on my woodlot. He then said, "I think you told me that there is not much you can do this early in spring, is that right?"

"You're right," I said. "I do a few things now in getting equipment cleaned up, charge small batteries for equipment, sharpen saws. Just the odds and ends to get going. But it's not a lot of time."

Dr. Brooks continued, "So what I thought is that you spend a minimum of four hours each day being occupied with cancer, the pain of it, your hot flashes, being awake at night, all of that. All that discomfort is related to the cancer. Even the additional time of getting dressed to get here is all related to coming for treatment. Is that true?"

"Yes, it is."

He said that was a lot of time to be thinking primarily about cancer and treatment. Many of the men who come to the center are employed, and very few of them travel as long as I did, so for them it is not their preoccupation. While they are concerned about cancer and affected by it, they then go off to a regular job and think about many other things besides coming here. And some men come very late in the day—after work. He said that for me, it's the opposite—cancer was the dominant part of my life.

He was quite convincing and ended his comments by asking, "See what I mean?"

I said, "Absolutely, yes, you're right, I hadn't even considered that." I nodded my head a moment and then said, "I listen to the radio on the way back and forth, and that's about it. Of course, I like to eat here because of the convenience and the food is fresh and healthy." I paused. "You're saying I should . . . what? Get some distraction of some kind, do some other things?"

"Well, that might help. It's not an easy answer. There's not much we can do about the basic time and effort you put into this; but, well, think about it. What other things might you do to get some diversion from cancer?"

I paused, and he waited for my response. "I guess it's true that even when I go home and am so tired that I have to take a nap, even though I resist it, that again is, like . . . well . . . as you say, all a part of the time spent on cancer. Yes, I have to take the nap because of the treatment. And then I get so mad since I can't get anything done."

"I understand that," Dr. Brooks said.

He then explained that most of the men who come to the center have a time when they collapse, either with some tears or major health complaints, some bitterness about the treatment, or maybe skipping a couple of days to avoid the daily concentration on cancer, even having some other illness come along.

He said, "A couple of men have just taken off a few days, which we don't recommend. We know that some have to do it. But this more serious upset that some other men have does not usually come until after the midpoint of treatment, and we watch for that possibility. Yours came at the beginning, and I'm still not clear how some other events contributed to your upset."

He looked at me for a moment and said, "That's why I am wondering how this amount of time that you spend going back and forth for cancer treatment, including other time that you think about cancer, was already having a strong influence on your general balance, your ups and downs."

"OK . . . ah . . . yes, I do agree with you." I was quiet for a moment, and my eyes began to well up as they seemed to do then when people expressed concern for me.

"Let me go over this with my family and see what I can do to change some of this," I said. I shrugged a bit, shaking my head slightly. "This is such a crazy problem."

I told him that I was now at the point where I just didn't have much energy for anything. I told him how tired I was and that I fought the naps because I was angry that I couldn't get anything done.

I added, "It's ridiculous, and I think, or I know I told you about this. I have fought the naps by walking around, going to the barn, and pushing myself to do things and to avoid lying down, even sitting down, but sitting upright. But yet, Elizabeth, the nurse at the other desk, and Suzanne too, told me that the way to protect my health is to take naps, because my body is demanding rest . . . demanding time to restore damaged tissues. And, of course, you told me the same."

He nodded his head in agreement. "Almost all men face the same problem, and remember you are also on hormone treatment, and that alone can reduce your energy. Your testosterone gets almost totally eliminated, and that's one of the major hormones that gives men energy and drive."

We were both silent for a few moments. Dr. Brooks began again.

"We want you to heal, and the way to do it is to rest when your body tells you to. What we say around here is 'Listen to your body.' That is the best sign or the best cue. Listen to your body."

He said that softly and firmly, and we looked at each other for a couple of moments.

As I felt a tiny bit of mist in one eye, I very gently nodded my head in agreement, thanked him, and we departed. As I drove home that day, I knew he was right. Cancer and its treatment had become the epicenter of my life.

In the coming weeks, I would have some diversions from preoccupation with cancer. Help would come primarily from my family, a neighbor, and two librarians.

CHAPTER 6

Dreams are often difficult to understand, and they have been interpreted probably as long as humans have conversed with each other. Sigmund Freud, the famous psychiatrist, called dreams the "royal road to the unconscious." They come from sources deep within us. When we make our own, we are at one and the same time the producer, writer, director, and the audience.

The dream that burst into my sleep early on Wednesday, March 13, 2003, during my first week of radiation, seemed to come from deep within me and was nothing that I or anyone would create for a pleasant diversion. It was about a possible violent death. It exhausted me and caused my weeping on the fourth day of treatment. It was in every way a nightmare.

The *Oxford English Dictionary* defines "nightmare"

> as a spirit or monster supposed to beset people and animals by night, setting upon them while they are asleep and producing a feeling of suffocation by its weight. [A nightmare is also] a feeling of suffocation or great stress felt during sleep, from which the sleeper vainly endeavors to free himself; a bad dream producing these or similar sensations.[11]

---

11. Oxford University Press, Walton Street, Oxford, London, 1971, 1926.

I have had only two nightmares in my life, at least during my adulthood. I have had many bad dreams, but nothing that has startled me awake, alarmed me, and made me apprehensive and irritable, followed by difficulty in achieving sleep again. Both of my nightmares were vivid and produced similar kinds of feelings the next morning and even throughout the day.

In the beginning of April 2003, I left a six-page letter at the nursing station for Dr. Brooks, describing what had happened prior to and on the fourth day of my radiation treatment. It included my analysis of what I believed was going on within me.

In the letter, I explained that there was more to the foundation for my upset than I originally thought and had told him. I then said that the letter was written for two reasons: to let him know what happened and also to help me understand myself better.

> On Sunday, March 9, the day before radiation started, I had just a
> half minute of quiet tears over feeling dependent on others. I had
> become aware of some short-term memory loss and found myself
> making a couple of computational errors as well as spelling errors.
> This was but a brief recognition that my mind was slipping, that
> I was forgetting how to picture words in my mind. I could always
> do that. To me, both those tiny events were serious.

I explained that this brief feeling of being dependent was probably related to some very caring comment that my son or daughter made to me now that I had cancer and was being treated for it. I believe I was weeping because of how much they care for me. I believe this related to a reversal of roles that I have been reluctant to accept. They now care for me in a parental way instead of the way I, as a parent, had cared for them.

I had always been quite accurate with adding large or multiple numbers, so it also bothered me to make errors. The spelling errors were probably much more significant, since I almost always won spelling bees up through the eighth grade, and my own family leaned on me often for word spelling.

With few exceptions, I rarely missed correct spelling. Now there was a clear hint that I was beginning to lose some of that accuracy.

> Later on March 9, my son, Peter; my daughter, Ingrid; and I took a family trip to Newton, Massachusetts, to see my other son, Kenneth, installed as the minister at the congregational church in town. This was a big event with various dignitaries in attendance, with flowing robes and colorful processions. At that same service, my only granddaughter, Isabelle, was baptized; and that was a joyous event. An emotionally powerful part of the service was the majestic music of Richard Strauss with five brass pieces and the full vibrant organ. My wife adored brass music, so I was wishing she were there not only to experience these important family and religious events but to also hear the clarity and strength of the music. Even the title of the prelude conveys the majesty: "Solemn Entry of the Knights of Saint John."

On Wednesday, March 12, I learned that my PSA had dropped from 7.6 to 0.15. I was elated, and my urologist was also quite pleased. I had pictured that it might rise slightly or decrease just a bit. I was in very good spirits, but that night I had extreme thrashing and restlessness, which is unusual for me even though I was now having hot flashes from the hormone therapy. I got about two hours' sleep in the morning. Just before waking, I had a dream that I was alone driving in a car in a beautiful parklike woods, wandering this way and that. I looked ahead and saw an absolutely beautiful area directly ahead that had many trees on a higher elevation, and I decided to drive there.

As I drove in that direction, I suddenly realized that I was starting down a steep hill. I became alarmed and was afraid of slipping down the hill and crashing into a deep ravine. I pumped the brakes very carefully and was just able to stop at the edge but was very frightened. Then I could see the drop of several hundred feet below and realized

I could have fallen on to the sharp rocks hundreds of feet below and been killed. The dream ended but was very vivid to me in the morning.

> The dream seemed to mean that I had been moving forward somewhat slowly into treatment. The symbolism of driving toward the higher ground was the good news of the lower PSA. But stopping at the edge of the cliff revealed my underlying worry and fear of dying from prostate cancer. My partially conscious fear of death was made clear to me in my panic that I could not stop from falling over the cliff. The dream also told me that just because I had a low PSA did not mean that I still could not die.

The dream suggests a number of possibilities—I am usually alone driving the car, so this is typical of my current life. The other possibility is that I would like to be in control of my medical care, or it may mean that I feel I am in control and yet that would be quite dangerous. I could definitely not only die from that but be killed in a painful way. Pumping the brakes suggests an earlier time in my life (before ABS systems), when I was quite independent—with no dependence on medical personnel.

I had tended to be almost dismissive of this disease. To friends I had referred to it as a garden-variety cancer, since so many men get it and so many recover. In one sense, I believed it to be less potent, especially when compared to other types of cancers and particularly breast cancer in women. I had not dwelled on the fact that men do die from prostate cancer. My greatest fear, which I admitted to myself quite readily, is that death from prostate cancer can be very painful when spread occurs into the pelvic and other bones; but then I denied that this would ever happen to me.

> On Wednesday morning, the twelfth, my daughter, who moved home temporarily while seeking new employment, left to go out of town for several days. On Thursday, March 13, the day of my upset, my son, Peter, who had driven me to the center the first

three days of radiation, left to go back to work. This meant that I drove to the center myself, and for some reason, I began to think about my wife and the times we drove together whenever either of us went for medical care. I became wistful, missing her, and some music on the radio reminded me of her. When I am reminded of her through music, I have feelings of pleasure. But this time I began to have tears of loss.

By the time I walked into the radiation area, I was feeling quite down, very alone, and depleted from almost no sleep on Wednesday night. Death was on my mind. When Andrea the therapist asked me how I was, I couldn't hold myself together and began to cry.

In summary, this was precipitated by several events: a brief feeling of dependency, a couple of elements of beginning decline from aging, a glorious day on Sunday with powerful music, an installation and baptism, my son and daughter leaving home about the same time, my beginning of radiation, good news about my PSA level, a vivid nightmare involving possible loss of control and a violent death, loneliness in thinking about my wife, and finally, the need for treatment as a dependent (patient role) in a hospital in contrast to my years-ago experience as a practitioner in two hospitals and several social and health agencies. It is surprising to me that so many events or activities could coincide at one time, but they did.

I explained that if I am in any way typical of persons with this illness, the possibility of death must be harbored frequently or constantly. It's much more clear to me now than before. This was a scary, scary dream. It was not something that a shower and a hot cup of coffee would erase or wash away. I thought about it before coming to the center and since starting radiation treatment, but my emotional connection to it had not yet occurred.

It was puzzling that a very positive PSA report could contribute to my upset. In looking back on that event, it is likely that the positive report could have muted the great fear and anguish in the dream. If the PSA had been as high as before treatment started, the dream could have been all the more frightening.

In the final paragraph of the letter, I wrote that I had been quite happy with all the care I received. I believed that the two therapists who served me thus far were expert and flawless as a team. I added that I couldn't say it much clearer than this: "When I drive to the hospital, I feel almost as if I am coming home to see my family."

CHAPTER 7

During the third week of my radiation, while I was lying on the table being pushed gently by Andrea and Sybil, another therapist, from one side to another to get me in the correct alignment with the cross beams of the red laser lights, I thought I would mention one of my concerns about myself since starting the radiation. I rather casually said that I noticed that I had gained a little weight recently.

Sybil, who was on my left, quietly and with obvious thoughtfulness said, "Oh, well, how much have you gained?"

I softly replied, "Oh, I'd say . . . about two pounds."

Andrea, on my right side, chipped in and asked, "Over what time period?" *Good questions*, I thought to myself.

They continued to push me from one side to another to align the tiny tattoos on my abdomen with the red laser lights.

"Well," I said, "it's two pounds, probably in, oh, the past five weeks."

The pushing on both sides stopped, as if by a prearranged, silent signal; and there was total silence in the room. Now this is a room that does not have a sound in it. No sound. None. There are no windows; it is a fully enclosed indoor room with a short hall to a secure door to prevent any type of radiation to escape. This is not just a subdued atmosphere. It's totally silent. Think death. And yet from this sudden short silence, there slowly emerged just the slightest squeak of a snicker, then a soft, muffled laugh, then a larger laugh, then both Andrea and Sybil laughing so that the entire process of preparing me for the radiation sequence totally ceased. They were both looking at me, simply laughing, and Sybil made the first comment.

"Listen," she announced with authority and firmness, although her voice contained a certain gentleness for my concern. "I can go out to dinner for the evening, and I can gain two pounds right then. Or more, *more*," she emphasized.

Andrea quickly added, "And do you know that I can walk into a bakery, take a long, deep breath, and gain at least two pounds?"

I looked from one to the other and joined in the laughter, realizing I was a bit unrealistic about presenting this as a concern; but while I could laugh at myself, it was a concern that I would continue to have. The three of us continued to snicker while they moved me around on the table.

"Well," I said, somewhat weakly, "I don't want to gain any weight. I've always been on the light side. Yes, but I see what you mean—that's not much; but I still would like to keep the same weight." For a few moments I smiled to myself and then almost laughed out loud as I thought about the comedian Rodney Dangerfield, whose standard line was "I get no respect around here."

And then in my mind, I adopted Dangerfield's view of himself and life. Here I am being treated for a serious cancer; I spill my guts about a health concern in a highly respected medical center to two of my most trusted new friends and professionals, and they laugh—yes, they actually laugh at me. Hey, I get no respect around here.

They returned to their task of aligning me on the table; the X-ray unit completed its work. Sybil and Andrea returned, and as I stood up and started dressing, Sybil commented that I certainly did not seem overweight. I had to agree, and she then said that I had given the two of them a good laugh.

The next day when I walked in and sat on the table, Sybil said that I had given her one of her best days here, since she laughed throughout the day in thinking about my two pounds. We began to talk about food again and how Andrea especially liked chocolate. Sybil didn't comment about this. This discussion was on Wednesday. On Friday, the cafeteria had a rich, decadent, double-layer chocolate cake for dessert; and I bought them a piece to share. On Monday, I discovered that they had both wolfed it down. Sybil also loves chocolate. My error was to buy only one slice.

*   *   *

Once a week, an appointment is made for all patients with the physician to whom each one is assigned. Routine checks are made of weight, blood pressure, blood oxygen flow, and other tests as needed. I was continuing to see Dr. Brooks, the oncologist who interviewed me in the beginning. Following the brief conversation with Sybil and Andrea, I thought I would bring it up with the nurse, Suzanne, who also had seen me for screening to the program. Upon inquiry, I said that I was doing OK, had no particular concerns, was feeling well, and had no abdominal problems. She checked my pulse and pressure, and while doing that I commented that I thought I had gained a little weight, and I didn't want to really gain any. She stopped what she was doing and looked at me.

"You—gaining weight?"

"Well, yes, a little bit." Here I thought I better be more specific. "Probably two pounds, maybe more in the past four to five weeks." I thought I better give all the data so she would have more information to evaluate.

I felt that she was looking at me as if I had just said that I was quitting the radiation program and I didn't care whether I died or not. I knew she was reaching for something to say. I guess it was a surprise for someone of my slight frame to express concern over excess weight. Well, she did have an answer, namely, that I didn't look in any way overweight, but that I could talk with Dr. Brooks about it when he came in. The thought in my mind when she left the room was that she was rolling her eyes.

Dr. Brooks came in a few minutes later; we shook hands, and he was friendly and cheerful, as he always seemed to be. He asked some of the basic questions about my radiation schedule, any change in my body that I could detect, and I assured him that all was well, that the time slot I had was quite acceptable, and it also meant that I could eat lunch here at the cafeteria occasionally, and that was a real convenience for me. I said to him, "Well, maybe this is a minor concern, but I gained a couple of pounds recently, and I don't want to gain any more weight."

His entire demeanor changed; there again was this look of disbelief, the same look that Suzanne gave me. Obviously she had not told him what I had said; maybe she wanted to let him have the full effect of this question without any time to prepare an answer. I offered the same data as before.

Well," he said, "that's not much weight to gain. And people do go up and down slightly with their weight."

I agreed but offered that I just didn't want to go on gaining weight. Brooks then obviously wanted to get a better grip on this question, so he asked whether I knew where on my body I had gained weight.

"Oh, I think it's probably around my waist," I said.

I quickly offered additional information. I told him I had never gained weight all my life—I've always been just about the same, except when I was aboard a minesweeper in World War II. We generally had good food, especially while at sea when we could catch fish, and we were fortunate to have a good cook. I had gone up to 138 pounds, and that was just too heavy for my frame, so I slowed down my eating and slowly reduced my weight. I had entered the navy at 120.

I said, "Let me explain a little more; maybe this will help." I cleared my throat for a second.

I explained that I've always been a small person. That's the way I see myself. In grade school, I was always the smallest boy in the room. In one way I hated it because other kids could pick on me, and I was not a good fighter. My father was only five feet two and ninety-two pounds, and we used to kid with him that he only weighed that when he was soaking wet.

I told him that my mother was also small, and somehow I got to be five feet seven. In WWII, I tried to join the coast guard because I enjoyed small boats. But the coast guard wouldn't take me because I was only five feet two; they wanted five feet six. So I went in the navy. I explained to him that it comes down to the simple fact that being thin is my identity. I am comfortable that way.

Then for a moment, I laughed. "One time when I was filling out a medical form and my wife was with me, she watched what I was writing. I put down 125 for my weight, which is what it was. She said, 'Why don't you put down 130? It looks a little better!' So I did."

I also told him that I didn't know I had knees until I was almost seventy. And even then, it didn't bother me that much. I had read that the knees give out sooner if someone is heavier. I've even talked with men in their fifties who have trouble with their knees. But I didn't even know I had arthritis in all my joints until I had one of those body scans, and my doctor told me I did. I added that I can still keep going and do physical work, and I don't have to take a lot of painkillers.

"So, I figure, well, maybe being lightweight isn't the worst," I said. "See what I'm getting at? Oh," I said suddenly before he had a chance to respond, "here's another amusing one. Remember I told you about the basal cell skin cancers I've had? Well, my dermatologist—this was about fifteen years ago—was removing for the third time a cancer on my chest. He and I had become friends; and as he was working on me, he suddenly said, 'Damn it, you're the skinniest patient I've ever had. You know that I'm cutting right now on your rib? There's just no skin left! But I'll get it pulled together.' And he did."

I paused.

"And right now I can't fit into my regular trousers, so I've had to buy pants with a 32 waist."

"So you see, I've never had to buy trousers, probably since I was age twenty-five, larger than either a 29 waist or 30 waist. And now I'm up to a 32, and that's just recently. So, well, you get the idea?" I looked at him.

"Well, I see what you mean about your childhood and early life. And there is truth about knees being painful with extra weight." He paused for a moment. "Thirty-two waistline, huh?"

"Uh-huh, yeah."

"Well, doesn't sound to me like that's awfully large."

There was another pause; and Dr. Brooks said, "Well, look, why don't you just drop your trousers for a moment and let's look at your waist."

He looked for a moment and said, "I don't see any problem here. Why don't we just watch it for a while and see what happens, but you look fine to me. But we do want you well nourished through this treatment, OK?"

As an afterthought, he added, "Remember, as people get older, some of the weight drifts down, if by gravity alone; muscles are not as taut as when we're younger and when we gain weight, as most people do as they age, then some of that weight will rest or reside in the waist area. And this weight may be nothing but increasing age."

Well, I thought to myself, *at least doctors have some objective criteria to evaluate a patient's condition. They can use concrete data and weigh (no pun intended) that information against the patient's self-description.* The look of puzzlement on his face had now totally disappeared. I thanked him for seeing me and for his comments, but I still walked out thinking that I'm not getting very far and not getting there very fast in relation to weight. I didn't know that in a couple of weeks, a new opportunity to discuss weight would become available.

*   *   *

Andrea, Sybil, and I talked a little bit about food from time to time: what would be in the cafeteria today, what we ate yesterday, and other idle chatter that occurred while another radiation session was to start. We talked about chocolate several times, and I mentioned a Thai restaurant in town where I found some interesting food. During one of those conversations, Sybil said, "You might want to talk with our dietician. Did you know that we have one here in the center?"

"Gee, no, I was not aware of that."

"She's not here every day, but it is quite easy to set up an appointment to discuss food and diets. Her name is Deborah; we're very fond of her, and she has helped many people here who are struggling with diets and upset stomachs, advising them about dietary changes during certain periods of treatment, many things like that. Patients really like her."

"I'd be pleased to meet with her," I said. "I worked at a public health agency for several years, and a nutritionist and I shared the same office. Therefore, we had a chance to talk about foods, diets, all those things. I learned a lot from her, and I was surprised at how little I knew about nutrition or diets. What should I do? Can you set up a time for me?"

"Absolutely," Sybil answered. "She's here three days a week, so how about Thursday after your session here if she's available at that time?"

"Sounds good to me."

"We'll confirm the time with her and check with you tomorrow. She'll come to the waiting room; it's an easy place to meet."

"Many thanks."

CHAPTER 8

Deborah arrived as planned. She was a petite woman, dark hair, neatly dressed, and her presence was in no way formal or official. Her manner was easy and open, and I found myself liking her very quickly. Her voice was soft, engaging. We chatted about incidental things as we walked to an office. It was easy to relate to her, and I thought she was expert in establishing a relaxed relationship rather quickly. But something else began to happen within me.

On a few rare occasions, my thoughts have been a bit romantic when meeting someone. This reaction is far more likely to happen when I listen to romantic ballads and lyrics. With some love songs, I have to sing along in my mind or may hum the tune softly. Today I did not understand what was happening to me, but I was far more interested in simply talking with Deborah, rather than talking about diets. My mind wandered a bit; and going through my head was the magic of an evening in a room where there is soft music, candlelight, couples dancing, wispy curtains moving in a gentle, warm breeze, bouquets of flowers on small tables, a small band playing, and a vocalist singing,

> Some enchanted evening, you may see a stranger, you may see a
> stranger, across a crowded room, and suddenly know . . . .

Reality broke this momentary spell. This was not a summer evening; it was a cold spring day. I had tired, scruffy boots on, not dancing shoes.

There was no magical soft light or music. It was late morning, and this was a hospital hallway, not a ballroom with soft light and lacy curtains. Flowers? Only on the hallway desk where volunteers sit. The woman who had charmed me was carrying a medical chart, leading me to a sterile, almost barren examining room. Poof, it was over.

Prior to our meeting and as we met, I had the thought that she would be sufficiently objective about nutrition and diet to take my thoughts about weight gain seriously. If I could get her on my side, then I could have others take my concerns seriously. I had never had to face weight increase before, and my experience in the navy was too far in the past to recall that I could simply slow down my eating, and for some reason, I did not think of such a simple solution. On the other hand, I was beginning to realize that my energy was diminishing; and food, especially high carbohydrate or rich food, is one way to store up and maintain some vigor and energy.

As we sat down, Deborah opened my chart to one of the first two pages and in the blink of an eye put her finger on one column at the top of the page. She did it very quickly and without a second's hesitation announced with apparent pleasure, "Oh good, you haven't lost any weight! We don't want that to happen. That's a problem when you're getting radiation." She didn't even look at me when she said it!

The emphasis in the first sentence was on the word "good"; and the gentle and measured force of her statement sounded as if she had finally, after weeks of examining me, discovered the sole source of all my problems. There was a finality to her statement. The three sentences together seemed like conclusive evidence that this would be the basis of our conversation.

My face must have looked just as blank as the doctor's and nurse's faces looked to me when I indicated my concern about adding a couple of pounds. I was so surprised at this instantaneous comment that I'm sure I didn't hear her next few sentences. If I heard them, I certainly did not comprehend them. I was dumbstruck; I had counted on the dietician being the key person to be on my side. After all, is there any adult in the United States who does not know that dieticians and nutritionists do not want people to gain too much weight? That was my reasoning. But her quick analysis of just one indicator of my experience at the center was weight, and don't lose any!

"Well," was about the best comment I could manage to make. "I . . . uh . . . well, that may be good, but I was . . . uh . . . you see, wondering about my diet or something since I thought I was gaining weight, and uh . . . well, you see . . . uh . . . I did ask Dr. Brooks, the oncologist, about this; but he didn't think, or I guess I should say, now how did he say it, oh, he thought, or maybe he said my weight was OK."

I was unable to put together a simple sentence.

"No, your weight is fine, and I'd like to see it go up a bit. Later on, you may not have much of an appetite; tell me, how's your appetite now?"

The preoccupation I was having with no support from Deborah on weight did not inhibit me from looking at her and suddenly realizing that she was a similar size as my wife, and her hands were small like my wife's and had what I believed were the same physical appearance. I now had the clear notion that she was a blend of many of my wife's friendly and warm characteristics with both interpersonal relationships and professional presence as well as some similar physical characteristics. This led me to a momentary disorientation, and I could not escape the initial perception of a very charming woman. No wonder that everybody liked her. I certainly did.

> There were birds on the wing, but I never heard them singing,
> No, I never heard them at all, till there was you . . . .

My feelings toward her were difficult to limit, but the reality of the clinical situation enabled me to begin to control those emotions.

Finally, I told myself to get all those thoughts out of my mind and concentrate on the discussion of food. Yet these feelings toward her were very strong. She was of the age when life can be in good balance. Probably middle to late thirties. Good years. I was immediately reminded of times that my wife and I danced together, whether out or at home. I especially remembered July 15, 1995, when my son was married. There was a five-piece combo, and my wife and I started dancing from the very beginning. We ended only when the band played the final piece, and that was after midnight and after all the young people had long since collapsed on the lawn outside.

"Umm, yes, it's OK, I don't have any problem with eating; and I've very seldom ever had problems with digesting food . . . uh, yeah, it's OK." I was definitely stumbling here, still off balance from the first couple of comments. Her question came to me so quickly that I was worried that I could not give a clear answer. I was still enamored by her skill and gentleness, but I was distraught that my greatest hope for a potential supporter had just evaporated within about twenty seconds of the time we sat down.

"Would you like to go over diet? We could go over a few things together if you think that would help," she said in an inviting way. "Oh," she interjected, "first, how are you doing generally with your treatment? Any special problems or concerns?"

"Uhh, not really, it's primarily the tiredness that comes with it; and I tend to take a nap once a day. That's a bit annoying since I don't get a lot done, but I understand it's one of things that happens with the radiation."

At that time, I felt far more negatively about the tiredness and hot flashes than the word "annoying" would convey, but I didn't want to say too much about that since the real focus of our meeting was to be about food.

"That's correct, and it is good to get rest when you can, and it's another reason that we like to know about your food intake. So maybe you can tell me about your diet."

"Hmm . . . ahhh . . . yes, what was it . . . oh . . . you said diet, well, sure let's do that."

By now I had caught my breath again, but I still felt like a swimmer about to drown when someone pulled me out and I could breathe again. I was now trying to think what I could say about diet that would be clear to her and be understandable for further planning. But I continued to be off balance from her similarity to my wife and my continuing interest in her rather than the discussion of diet.

"OK," she observed, "you are almost in your fourth week, with five more to go after that. You say you're having no trouble eating, but tell me a bit about what you eat."

Finally, I firmly removed myself from these very pleasant, albeit brief, feelings of deep affection. I rejected any further romantic thoughts. I told myself emphatically to stop looking at her. At the same time, I was glad to have thoughts about my wife. I began to differentiate clearly between Deborah and my wife, but the similarities remained close; it was very disconcerting. This was totally different from the experience we all have of meeting someone and then saying later, "She really reminds me of . . ." My experience was far more intense, more surprising, and certainly more satisfying.

While I was still baffled over what was happening to me, the trancelike experience faded away and was over. I concentrated on diet.

I told her that my daughter, Ingrid, lived with me, and she usually prepared meals, and I often helped in preparation; it sort of depended on what we were having. We usually ate different breakfasts, and our schedules were also different except when she came with me to the center. She had also been getting some medical treatment here in town, but she sometimes wanted to drive me, simply because I was sometimes rather tired and she wanted to help me. I really appreciated that. I went into a brief description of breakfasts.

"I add fruit in season; but most often it includes a half or more of banana, lunch of a sandwich or something left over from dinner the night before, often some soup, sometimes homemade, also homemade pea soup, bean soup with a ham base. Supper includes a small piece of meat, often chicken, and increasing amounts of fish, but very little red meat or white potatoes. We have fresh salads, and the vegetable is often the eternal and never-ending broccoli. We also eat soy products. About once a week, I'll eat eggs for breakfast. We also use low-fat cottage cheese, low-fat yogurt, no-fat or 1 percent milk; that's about it. Oh yes, and we've also been eating some more nuts since they have some good nutrients in them."

"How about desserts after dinner or snacks in the evening?"

"Oh yes," I stumbled. "If Ingrid makes something, such as a cake or some cookies, usually low fat and low sugar, I'll have some of that; but dessert is not a regular event. I occasionally make rice pudding. Before bedtime, I may have a small glass of hot milk, especially in the winter. I avoid all other fluids in the evening, since that would awaken me, and I have enough of that with my hot flashes."

"Eat ice cream?"

"No, I just don't use it. Well, I shouldn't say that; I'll have a small amount when my son comes home periodically, but that's about all. It's sort of just enough to taste it, but there's always ice cream in the house. There was one point in my life when I had almost no ice cream for many years."

"Really?"

"Yes, but I just didn't eat it."

"Don't like it?"

"Uh, no, but it isn't that good for you, well, you know about that . . . too much fat, too much sugar. Oh, and of course there is good protein in ice cream. But I will eat it on occasion if I'm with a group of people who are having some."

"Eat other rich things?" she asked.

"Not that often, but sure I'll occasionally splurge on something, but I'd just as soon not."

"Well," Deborah said. Her tone suggested an end to that part of the discussion. And as soon as she said that, I knew the pitch was coming my way.

"I think it would be good for you to start to eat a few heavier and a few richer foods, but not too many. Your diet, as I understand it, is a bit on the lean side—and that's good, quite good, for a well-balanced meal; but right now with your treatment here, I'm going to suggest that you change some of your food intake." She paused. "You know what comfort food is?"

"Sure, it's, uh . . . mashed potatoes and gravy, pancakes, maple syrup?"

"Right. You like french fries?"

I didn't respond since she went on to suggest that I stay with the fresh vegetables—they are important—but for now, at least for a little while, eat some of the foods that Americans have all been eating for a long time and may not have been the best for us nutritionally. That's the food I would need now and through the rest of the treatment. She reminded me that the oncologist had told me that in the latter part of radiation, I would be more uncomfortable. Some days I might not feel like eating.

She emphasized, "You may feel like eating, but we don't want you to then drop too much weight during that time. You will be tired enough."

She added that protein would be important for the rest of the radiation program, and even beyond that. Deborah noted that it takes as much time to recover from the problems related to radiation treatment as it has taken to provide the radiation. So it would be essential after the end of treatment to eat a diet that maintained my weight and energy to help my body recover. Good protein, whether it is from red or white meat, plus many other sources of protein, is vital. The treat foods, like pie, a little ice cream, were OK now and then since they are recognized as special treats.

She then started to add some other changes that dismayed me.

"I'm going to suggest that you not only eat more meat but you might even choose some with a little bit of fat, not much—you understand?"

"Really?" I was almost going to challenge her on that one.

"Yes, it's all right just for this time of treatment. Go to 2 percent milk, whole cottage cheese, and whole-fat yogurt. That will help to maintain you until you get beyond all the effects of the radiation. How many days of radiation will you have?"

"Ah, forty-three."

"Well, then that is eight and a half weeks. So, just to emphasize, it's best for you to stay on this different diet to make sure you hold your weight and keep nourished well beyond the time you stop here. And you might also have some weight gain from the inflammation in your abdomen. That happens fairly often from the radiation."

I breathed quietly, saying nothing, now trying to take all of this in. It was the opposite of the way I had been living for a good number of years. After a few moments, I said, "OK, that all seems clear to me." She smiled in return.

My life was changing fast. I didn't especially like what I was hearing, but I did like the thought of eating some of those richer foods again.

Our meeting was essentially over. I thanked her and said, "I'll change my food habits and get back to you and let you know how it's going. I did read all the materials handed out when I started here, but I guess I just didn't connect on changing anything about meals. I wasn't aware of how diet would be so important."

She wished me well and said she would be glad to see me again. If Deborah found me a little disconnected in the meeting, she was right. I was quite distracted by how much she resembled my wife. While this bothered me, I was also content that I could think about some pleasant times with my wife.

I was so baffled and so troubled by the strong romantic feelings I had toward Deborah that I never described them to anyone. Never.

We met two or three times later while passing in the hallways and would do a very quick review on food changes. I let her know that my family doctor had totally supported her recommendations. Dr. Shah, my physician, also reminded me that food is far more than nutrition; it is a social and family event, and it should also bring pleasure. Deborah was pleased to learn of her support. When we talked in the halls, I did not have the strong feelings experienced in the first meeting. Nevertheless, I was quite pleased to talk with her.

*   *   *

Shortly after I arrived home and before I planned to collapse on the sofa, Ingrid walked into the kitchen; and I said, "Guess what?"

"Oh?"

"You remember I told you I was going to meet with the dietician? Well, she and I talked for more than a half hour. She was a delightful person, but I'm not sure I liked what she said. You know what she said? I have to start eating more 'comfort food,' like mashed potatoes and gravy and . . ." I couldn't even finish the sentence.

"I told you, I told you. That's what you should start eating; you need more of those richer foods because of what's happening to your body. You should listen to me first. I told you that. Do you remember? And just remember, I said it before the dietician said it. Now maybe you'll believe me!"

"All right, all right, all right," I pleaded. "I'm guilty; you were right. I should have listened. So I guess we have to change my diet a bit."

CHAPTER 9

In later months, I thought several times about my reaction to the meeting with Deborah, the dietician. But many months later, I began to wonder about all of the feelings that had emerged from within me. Because of a range of mood changes and occasional crying that I found myself having as well as experiences of feeling emotional changes without clear stimuli, I began to realize that there was something artificial, or something distinctly different, about the level of my response to Deborah. In one respect, why shouldn't I have extra friendly feelings in response to meeting someone who represented, in several ways, my wife of forty-seven years?

But would my feelings have been so strong, or so sudden, without some distinct changes within me? My response was in a small way directed to Deborah, but my genuine feelings were in relation to my wife. I checked a few of my earlier notes and was reminded of how quickly my body had changed following the beginning of hormone therapy. I was also being influenced by both the strength of, and the consequences of, the radiation treatment.

These feelings were all out of character for me. I probably did not dwell on them too much, since I was far more concerned about my determination to continue with the treatment, to cope with my lack of energy, with my tiredness, and what I considered to be severe hot flashes.

The first injection of the hormone to diminish or destroy the testosterone was on December 11, 2002. In less than a month, I was having intense and continuing hot flashes. I would awaken at night with extensive hot flashes; the worst night was when I was awakened six times and was totally exhausted for most of the next day. One evening in early February 2003, I took off my sweater, then my shirt, then stood outside on the back step in my undershirt at five degrees below zero for three minutes and finally cooled down. Both my son and daughter saw this episode.

There were many other times that I stood on the back porch in my T-shirt that winter. In a later letter to Dr. Donovan, my second urologist, I described myself as looking like a cormorant bird on the Maine coast with its wings held out in a horizontal position to dry off.

Dr. Tyson, my urologist at the time of the first two injections, suggested that I switch on the next visit to a three-month injection, rather than the one-month shot. On February 6, 2003, I sent him a letter expressing concern over taking a three-month shot. I was fearful about having too much of the powerful Lupron Depot in my system at once, even though it is time released.

In the second paragraph of that letter I said,

> The daytime ones [hot flashes] are easier to respond to, but the nighttime flashes are beginning to deplete me. I have had two nights of five wake-ups and two nights of four wake-ups. Three seems to be an increasing pattern. This is not a complaint, but a description. Perhaps this response to the Lupron is totally normal.

I also referred to my general overreaction to medications, citing a mild prescription I had received from Dr. Shah and had to discontinue within ten days because it made me so sluggish. What I had not said to Dr. Tyson was my question of why the injection was not calibrated according to body weight. I later directed that question to Dr. Donovan, my other urologist.

It was apparently a one-size-fits-all concoction, but I still question why a person at 130 pounds gets the same injection as a person at 260 pounds.

I understood that the hormone to suppress testosterone might also alter moods as well as help to kill cancer. It was this mood alteration, I believe, that contributed to my increased response toward Deborah. That specific response, although I believe it was recognized only by myself, nevertheless caused me personal embarrassment and made me question whether I might be responding strangely or inappropriately to other persons in social situations. In addition, altered moods may contribute to erratic or unpredictable behaviors, as well as to errant decisions. I don't think this happened to me, but I slowly became more concerned about poor judgment in making decisions.

Still later I decided to go with the three-month injection; but this did not, in my mind, significantly change my emotional balance more than I had already experienced. My decision to take the three-month injection was partly based on the fact that I was very tired and could avoid driving to more medical appointments. I also knew that I could return to the once-a-month injections.

Confirmation of these mood changes also came from Dr. Brooks, my oncologist, and from my personal physician, Dr. Shah, since they both observed my mood swings and discussed them with me during the nine weeks of radiation and even after that. They were certainly better observers of my moods than I was.

Dr. Shah offered me medication to smooth out the "ups and downs," as she described them. She also used the word "leveling." The oncologist referred to smoothing out my alternating moods. I became slowly aware that I had some of the changes that were, in a sense, like a very short bipolar disorder. However, they were not as severe in either direction, and they were not as long standing. At least, that was my perception.

Clear evidence of my increased sensitivity to both the hormone therapy and the radiation is in the frequency of tears that I had, sometimes with no apparent external reason. They could emerge from any random thoughts I might have; but they often resulted from very positive, caring, or thoughtful comments that friends or relatives might make to me or from powerful classical music, from thinking about my wife, or from romantic or religious music, and from romantic lyrics. They also could begin when I might be tired, or very tired of feeling tired and wiped out, or when I wished I could get something accomplished but I didn't even have the energy to start. Several days when I came home from the center, I would put my head down on the table or sit on the sofa and simply cry, for what seemed to me no apparent reason. But I never shed tears like that before the two treatments began, nor several months after they ended.

The event with Deborah was difficult for me to fathom, and only in retrospect from a distance of many months could I begin to place these several events together and understand that I had experienced strong emotional changes. I knew the internal physiological reactions, primarily hot flashes, that I was having to the new hormone. But I was unable until later to recognize how significantly the hormone also affected my perceptions and my moods.

The impressive unrelenting power of hormone therapy, in this instance the injection of Lupron Depot, is suggested in the pharmaceutical company statement about this medication, technically called leuprolide suspension.[12] During a twenty-four-week treatment phase with fifty-six patients, it was found that in the first week of treatment, serum testosterone increased by 50 percent in the majority of patients. But serum testosterone dropped to the castrate[13] range "within 30 days of the initial depot injection in 94 percent (51 of 54) patients for whom testosterone suppression was achieved." Within sixty-six days, it had dropped in all fifty-four patients. It is no wonder that a patient's moods, feelings, and even behavior may be altered so quickly and so extensively.

[12.]   Clinical Studies Section, TAP Pharmaceuticals, Inc., Lake Forest, IL 60045, USA, by Takeda Chemical Industries, Ltd., Osaka, Japan, 541.

[13.]   Meaning the equivalent of surgical removal of the testicles.

It was the internal reactions that I would refer to at a later time as "the stranger within me." Still later I would realize reduced muscle mass and decreased physical strength. I believed that the hormone totally subordinated me to its unique power. I hated it because I believed it changed me into someone I had never been and someone I did not understand.

The event with Deborah could be considered a "high," and it was in marked contrast to my depressed upset on the fourth day of radiation, as described earlier. The latter was certainly an extremely low point, and I simply could not understand what was happening to me. I was totally baffled about my sadness and crying. A mental health clinician might have called it a transient mood disorder, since it was of rather short duration. That event certainly had clear stimuli, but was my response normal, or was it an overreaction? In examining both of those events now from a distance in time, I believe that both of them represented significant examples of the opposite ends of my newly expanded emotional range.

As I thought about the changes I felt, I wondered how atypical my behavior might have been. I wondered again how a mental health clinician might view the mood changes. I decided to look at the *Diagnostic and Statistical Manual,* a standard reference work for mental health professionals. Clinicians use this volume to help them assess the presence, features, and extent of a mental disorder. Since "mood disturbance" is a recognized side effect of the combination of radiation and hormone therapy, I selected that section of the manual.

The major feature of this change—or this behavior—is the "significant distress or impairment in social, occupational or other important areas of functioning." It includes a

"1. depressed mood or markedly diminished interest or pleasure in all, or almost all, activities, and

2.   an elevated, expansive or irritable mood."[14]

---

14.   American Psychiatric Association, *Diagnostic and Statistical Manual of Mental Disorders,* 4th ed., Text Revision, Washington, D.C., 2000, 400–410.

A third requirement is that the patient must have no other category of organic or psychological disorder. The final feature for using this assessment requires that if there are medical reasons that caused the disorder, then that precipitant must be included in the diagnosis.

My behavior was episodic, not continuous, and not as intense as in number 1. I displayed an irritable mood many times, but I was not unusually expansive. My behavior fell into no other area of mental disorder. Therefore, I believe that my mood variations could best be diagnosed as a "transient mood disorder precipitated by hormone and radiation treatment."

One other very small event is an example of my highs and lows. Three days after I wept on day four of the radiation, as Andrea and I were walking into the radiation room, she asked, "And how are you today?" Before she asked, I believe she could see that I was OK.

"I'm kicking high today," I responded. "So let's both kick high together—ready?"

Whereupon I threw both arms straight out to my sides and kicked my right leg straight out and up as far as it would go. Andrea did the same, and we laughed together. When we entered the radiation room, Sybil was there, and the three of us did the same kick.

An example of a brief, sudden low occurred on April 3, 2003, almost four weeks into radiation treatment. I was having a very pleasant lunch with a friend from a nearby college. We conversed about a wide range of subjects, and then rather suddenly I began to get tears in my eyes, and as before, I did not know what was happening to me. Some tears ran down my face. We stopped talking, and I wept softly for about two minutes. I was sad, but I recovered quickly.

I didn't know it at the time, but I would soon have still another very low episode, the lowest, most angry, and most bitter I was to have during the entire radiation regime. My personal physician, Dr. Shah, would patiently help me through my rage.

A final example shows the intensity of my emotional trajectory. Just before completing the radiation, I wanted to express my appreciation to all the cancer center staff members who served me. Having written parodies of musical lyrics and some simple poetry in the past, I decided to try a poem. I asked my neighbors Charlotte, a librarian and extensive reader, and her husband, a successful editor, to listen to it. They agreed, and we sat in their living room. I was pleased with what I had written and was reading it smoothly in the beginning, and then I began to feel the emotion in it, and I had to pause a couple of times.

As I reached the last six lines or so, I started to cry, paused a longer time, dried my face, then pulled myself together very slowly and finished it. I apologized; they said no apology was needed. They knew I was having a difficult time with treatment. I believed I could read a simple poem of thanks directed to cancer staff to two neighbors in the privacy of their home. I wasn't even capable of that. This happened on Sunday, four days before my last day. I was the weakest ever in terms of physical and emotional depletion. Of greater importance here is the fact that I was completely unable to recognize how fragile I had become.

Some months later, the three of us were talking about serious illness and its effects upon one's balance. Charlotte said that during my treatment, I seemed to be more "fragile" than before. I reacted to situations in a more distressed way; I also seemed more intense. She recalled my unusually sad response to the illness of a neighbor. She perceived my responses as much greater than I otherwise would have. In contrast to that change, she observed that I was also very determined, almost rigidly determined, about my driving to and completing the cancer treatment.

It was these highs and lows, the strength of them, their unpredictable character, and my apparent difficulty in both understanding and handling them, that I referred to in a thank-you poem to the center staff when radiation was over. I had written the lines during the last week of treatment. As I now read them two years later, I can see that I could not understand the surges within me; I could not separate one from the other. But I could define the external symptoms. I certainly could not control their arrival or departure, nor how long they would possess me. I was a victim of their exploitation. Tragically, I had no ability to differentiate one from the other and no personal defenses against such newly formed powers. Parts of the poem[15] state,

Where emotions, confused and bizarre reside . . .

To yield to alien hormones, restless, unruly . . .

You were the anchor when my spirits flagged low, and you laughed with me when my spirits soared . . .

You were steady when I faltered.
You were sure, reassuring when I could never be sure.

These all reveal my awareness of the roiling emotions within me, the large ups and downs that I felt at that time. Only in looking back after the passage of considerable time could I see more clearly the pattern of changes and see more clearly how specific highs and lows played out. While I knew what I felt, I could not grasp their identity, or the extent of their power over me; and I had no prior experience in managing these complex wide-ranging forces.

As much as I resented the several changes in me, I continued to be thankful for these alien hormones, since they helped to control the cancerous growths. As I look back on this treatment experience, it was not too high a price to pay for my recovery.

---

[15]   The complete poem is in chapter 13.

CHAPTER 10

Passing the halfway mark of radiation was a rewarding moment. However, this midpoint is partly an illusion, since I was halfway there in terms of time, but not the full buildup of radiation treatment. When radiation is complete, then the patient is halfway there. Treatment benefit is highest on the last day of treatment, but hormone treatment continues at full power. In addition, an equal number of days are required to recover from the assault of radiation as it takes to give the radiation. So the power of the accumulated radiation continues. Nevertheless, there is the psychological achievement of being halfway there, and that gave me a boost of energy.

Many changes occurred starting during the fourth and fifth weeks of radiation. One day I noticed my beard in the mirror and was puzzled that I did not need a shave. I recalled that I had last shaved over thirty-six hours ago. I usually have to shave every day in order to look neat, although I often left it go for several days when working at home, especially when in my woodlot. I watched the growth of beard for a week's time and confirmed that I did not need to shave as often. I then recalled what I had been told and also read in the cancer booklets[16] about hair loss. I realized that the hormone therapy had caused this change. My hair was either diminishing in growth or falling out.

Soon I became aware of other changes I learned to expect. This included loss of hair under the arms, chest, abdomen, lower arms, and upper and lower legs. One of the literature handouts noted that "pelvic hair" would diminish, and I discovered that the term "pelvic" also included the term "pubic." Why couldn't they say "pubic?" That's a bit more specific. That was the last hair to leave, and since I had lost almost all the other hair on my limbs and body, I just shrugged my shoulders and said, "Oh, so what, it doesn't make any difference any more." Of minor interest was that I lost no hair on top of my head, but I had already lost most of that hair years ago.

My upper arms very clearly lost muscle volume, and I know I was less strong than before. Part of that loss may also have been due to lack of exercise and use of upper body muscles. This loss bothered me more than loss of hair, but I also realized that the hair would return, and I expected to be active again and recover muscle strength.

During this entire period, I was exceedingly tired, and my body demanded rest. One day I napped for two hours, and that made me very angry. But there was little I could do about my weariness. I had always counted on a morning shower to help me wake up. But during this time especially, a shower did nothing for me. It was a waste of time. A waste of water. A waste of my limited energy. I felt just as drugged and weary after a shower as before. I began to wonder why I should even take one, except for cleanliness.

In the latter part of radiation, I began to have pain during urination. It was difficult to start the flow as well as pain in starting it. I wished I

[16.]　*What You Need to Know about Prostate Cancer*, National Institutes of Health, Public Health Service, U.S. Department of Health and Human Services; *Prostate Cancer: What It Is and How It Is Treated*, Zeneca Pharmaceuticals, 1993; *Radiation Therapy and You*, National Cancer Institute, Public Health Service, U.S. Department of Health and Human Services.

didn't have to start, but there was no choice. The word "burning" was never sufficient for me; I had in mind the word "sizzling," as in pieces of sausage in a saucepan throwing droplets of fat in the air. That's how exceedingly hot urination felt to me, especially when trying to start the flow. I was given a prescription for Flomax.

Flomax or Maxflo, what's the difference? The pharmaceutical writers did not have to think long to construct that name. It explained everything, and it was somewhat helpful. The additional problem at this time was the pressure to urinate. At one point, I got almost a handful of urine when I had to use a rest stop on the way home. There were many other close calls. During this latter period of treatment, I had selected four places along the trip where I could use a bathroom. I had to stop several times even though I was always careful to use a bathroom prior to leaving from or returning home.

The center staff told me that defecation could be quite uncomfortable during this time, since feces would be fragmented from the cumulative power of the radiation. The radiation "spray" strikes the bowel tissue and waste material just as it strikes the prostate gland. I faced the same problem of starting a bowel movement as in starting urination. It hurt so much that I dreaded using the toilet, but again what choice is there? At least I did not have diarrhea, as many men get.

But the increased bowel movements meant increased sensitivity, and there was frequent bleeding. I also developed hemorrhoids that added to the pain. I then had to use two over-the-counter medicines to soften and heal the anal area. At that time, I had reduced almost all fibrous foods from my diet. The handout literature I was given also said that light burning of the abdominal skin might occur, since the radiation beams obviously have to go through the skin. I experienced no sunburn of any kind.

CHAPTER 11

In early 2001, I had been receiving medical care from an internist in a group practice, and my doctor left to work elsewhere. I was concerned about this; and my friend, Denise, a nurse in the organization, let me know that two new doctors, a husband and wife, would arrive shortly. Maya Shah, MD, was not only a board-certified internist, but she had a special interest in dermatology. For me, that was a stroke of luck, since I grow a ready supply of skin cancers. Whenever one is removed, another quickly seems to takes its place. Dr. Shah, I would discover, never lets one escape.

Denise had told me that the existing staff was very pleased about the arrival of this couple, and she believed I would be very happy with Dr. Shah. I was waiting in the examining room for a regular appointment; and this very cheerful and attractive woman, dressed in lovely but also businesslike clothing, stepped in and shook my hand and introduced herself. I expressed my pleasure in meeting her. She stated that she had looked at my chart and then reviewed all parts of it with me for a few minutes, describing all that she had observed about me.

I was surprised that she had read virtually every page of my record. She explained some of my health characteristics that she would want to follow and added that she would be glad to attend to the skin problems. There was no need to ask any questions since she seemed to have covered everything. I couldn't have been more pleased, and my initial impression of her competence and warmth was borne out by her later care of me, especially during the cancer treatment.

When I saw Denise a short time later, I said, "Denise, I just had my first meeting with Dr. Shah. I just couldn't believe it. She is marvelous. I liked her in the beginning and the way she presented herself. By the middle of the meeting, I was totally impressed with her skill and manner; and by the end of the meeting, I felt very fortunate to have her as my physician."

Denise nodded her head in a positive way and replied, "I just knew you'd like her."

In the late fall of 2004, I saw Dr. Shah's husband on the street and introduced myself to him, describing how totally helpful she has been to me. I added that I liked her from the minute I met her.

His immediate response, including a broad smile, was, "I felt exactly the same way when I met her."

*　　*　　*

I had met with Dr. Shah twice during the period approaching and the beginning of the radiation treatment. My next meeting with her was on April 24, 2003. I had a little more than two weeks of radiation ahead. I was really down, very tired, generally anxious, and a bit irritable. I was not turning any of my annoyance on other people; I was really angry over what was happening to me.

By this time in the treatment regime, I was still going through considerable discomfort with bowel difficulties, some rectal bleeding, problems in urinating, moodiness, and then crying on occasion at home and at the center. I was up every night between three or four times, always awakened by the hot flashes, and then I had trouble getting back to sleep.

The meeting started off slowly, but I rather quickly began to describe my tiredness. I probably didn't even ask how she was at the beginning of the meeting, for I was so preoccupied with my weariness.

"I'm tired, I'm so tired, and now I'm tired of being tired. I am so damned tired of being tired."

I started to weep slowly then began to weep openly and express bitter comments about what I was experiencing.

"I'm exhausted, I'm absolutely exhausted, and I'm so tired of it. I sleep, but my sleep is broken—I'm up every night three to four times with the hot flashes. Once I was up six, six times. Then I can't squirt right away. I have to wait, then it comes, and it hurts, it's hot, it burns, it feels terrible. And now when I have a bowel movement it hurts. I dread having to empty my bowels. I have to, but it hurts so much that I fear doing it. And then I've been bleeding when I do have a movement. But," and then I groaned, "I knew these things could happen; it's in all the brochures."

I told her how, after getting up at night, I flopped back in bed and couldn't get to sleep. Or I crawled back, or just dragged myself back to bed. When I awakened, I felt drugged, didn't know what time it was, often didn't care.

I told her that I didn't know why I couldn't take this, why I couldn't endure it, but I couldn't. Then I would reverse myself and say that I could. Then I angrily contradicted myself, sighed, and said, "But I really can't. I'll be so glad when this damn thing is over, so glad . . . sooo . . . glad."

I described how the hot flashes come so often. In the daytime, you could do something, take off a sweater, a shirt, cool down. I didn't know what a person would do in summer with these damn things. I didn't know how women could put up with them. I told her again that all of this was so damn tiring.

Dr. Shah was silent; she just listened to me.

I told her that at night it was a pain, maybe worse than day. I always put on a pajama top, because I slept in a cool room. But then I would have to throw it off, and I would sometimes say to it, "Get the hell off of me," and throw it as far away as I could. I explained that I tore the shoulders on two of them because I almost ripped them off my back.

I paused and took a couple of breaths. "You know, when I read all that stuff about what would happen during treatment, I figured, 'So what, I can handle that.' But reading it and experiencing it are two different things . . . totally different."

I paused again to blow my nose, clean my face, and take a few breaths. I realized the tears were coming down my face, dropping off my chin as I leaned forward. She handed me another tissue, and I welcomed it. I was not ashamed to weep in front of her. I felt no dependence, no shame by accepting a tissue. By this time I was aware she was patting me softly on the knee, which I found to be very comforting. Then I started again, this time on dependence.

"And then I cry at the center once in a while; well, I maybe, I should say it's not too often. I don't even know how many times I cry," I explained softly.

"Just as I did the other day. I am so embarrassed, but they don't seem to mind. They accept it, but I don't accept it. I am also totally humiliated to walk with red eyes, often with tears still moist on my face through a hallway where both staff and other patients can observe me. It's embarrassing, I hold my head down.

"But here"—I paused to breathe a moment—"here's the thing that really . . . really gets me." For emphasis, I slammed my fist on the desk to my right. The desk surface was hard, but my fist was just as hard. Then I raised my voice; it too was rigid and firm.

"I hate it, I hate it, I absolutely hate it when I cry in front of center staff and they offer me tissues to wipe my face. I'm the one . . . I *am* the one who used to hand out the tissues to people as they cried; I was the one in that seat," I said, pointing to hers. "I used to hand them out, and now they're handing them out to me. It makes me furious. I was . . . I was the one," I emphasized, "who interviewed people; I was the one who helped them with problems."

My speech became faster as if to emphasize that I had told parents about medical findings on their child, I helped them in planning for further treatment, and I listened to them, and when they cried, I opened the drawer here and gave them tissues, and now they were giving tissues to me. I was the strong one; I was the one who listened. "Damn it," I said, "I just can't take it, can't take it, I cannot, I cannot," I burst into a flood of tears again.

I wept bitter tears then clenched my teeth. My body rested slightly. I was quiet for a moment, breathing slowly to catch my breath, almost hoping that by breathing I could get rid of this pain, this hurt, this damn dependence, this seeming reversal of fortune that I hated, hated. She continued to hold her hand on my knee, sometimes giving a small pat.

"I am . . . so . . . damn . . . mad . . . about being dependent. I just can't handle that. It's the one thing I cannot endure. I don't know why I can't handle it." I shook my head slowly back and forth as if to indicate how totally confused I had become.

I became quiet again, wiping my face, wondering why I had not gone into total hyperventilation with the loss of breath from crying and then the deep inhalation to recover. I didn't look at her with my outrage; I knew that she was attentive and cared. In one sense, it did not matter whether she spoke or not.

Dr. Shah was there, and that was all that mattered; she never tried to slow me down, never tried to suggest that all would change, never dismissed anything I said, no matter how outrageous, no matter how selfish, no matter how infantile I was in my beliefs. How could I dare to believe that I was so special, so entitled, so privileged that I did not have to face pain during treatment as others do?

I told her again how much I hated it when they offered me tissues. I told her softly, and this time more reflectively, how much I hated being dependent. I still wanted to be the strong one—to stand by, to let a client weep, to let the tears happen, to give quiet reassurance. I paused after that declaration and said, "And here I am, just look at me."

There was sadness in my voice, but the tone still conveyed the sharp edge of anger that some great, immense injustice had been done to me.

Absorbed, totally absorbed in myself, I ended these stormy and self-critical comments with, "So now it's me . . . so . . . now it's me, so now I'm the one who cries. I'm the one," I said in total resignation of what I had become. "Now . . . it's . . . me."

*   *   *

I did not want sympathy; I was simply bitter about this turn of events in which I believed the tables had been totally turned on me. I needed her to hear me out, to listen. She did, and she did not have to say anything, to do anything. I didn't ask for answers, because I knew there were no easy answers. I was being forced by strong emotion to remove, to rid myself of this pain. Any answers would have to come from within me, not from someone else, would have to come from my acceptance of being a patient. I was no longer a practitioner; I had to assume the patient role, with all the changes that entails. The answers for me were not in an injection, not in a pill, not in a capsule. They were inside me.

I carried the practitioner role for years. I had had few illnesses in my life; my two times in the hospital for "fake" heart attacks were very short and not painful, not stressful in any way. But the constant radiation treatment here was intense, crushing, constantly assaulting; and the hormone therapy, that damned "stranger in my body" as I called it, was equally debilitating in the way it altered my feelings, my sleep, and my moods.

The elimination of testosterone took the hair off my body, reduced my beard, shrunk my genitals, shrunk my muscles, confused me, made me irrational, weakened me all over, and even distorted my very self-definition. In fact, the hormone that changed me was no longer a "stranger in my body," but the stranger had become me. I was no longer the person that I had known all my life; I now was—that is, I, my very self—had become this stranger that I detested. *I was the stranger.* I wished I could vomit, vomit to get this repulsive, writhing, controlling, manipulating serpent expelled from my body.

So, by any measure whatsoever, I was very mixed up. I was getting good medical care, but I didn't fully comprehend that I was a patient, definitely a patient and would have to start acting like one.

I sat there beside her depleted, empty, continuing to look down at the floor, taking short breaths, taking another tissue. My body felt hot, drained of strength. I felt limp. I got all these burning, emotionally searing feelings out that had been residing, brewing inside me for too long. After a few more quiet moments, we began to talk, reflecting in subdued tones on the volume and intensity of hate and condemnation that I had just directed on myself and what was happening to me. I then began to have some sense of the extent of energy I had just expended, the amount of physical strength that I had used to express this pain, even though I was sitting in a chair the whole time.

I understood my depletion a little better when I very slowly sat back in the chair and could feel my muscles become less taut, my shoulders and arms droop a bit, my torso sink slightly into the chair, and my shoulder blades slowly touch the back of the chair. I could feel the moistness in my body. My face felt enlarged, very warm. There was sweat on my forehead.

I never complained that she gave me tissues; I was never mad at her or mad that she gave them to me freely. I placed her in an entirely different category of care. She was, in my mind, totally on my side, whereas those at the center were somehow different. They knew me in a different way, but I'm not sure how. I was ashamed to weep before them but never embarrassed or fearful of what I might say to, or reveal to, Dr. Shah. She would understand no matter what. But for the others, I would have to hold back any and all tears, defend my tears, deny them, deny, avoid any dependency.

I said to her slowly, reflectively, "I do like all the staff members at the center. They are all very kind to me . . . and to all other patients. They are extremely kind." I said softly, "I have even had moist eyes a number of times because they are so considerate in things they say, in their gestures . . . in . . . everything they do."

I shook my head a little and added, "In spite of that, I don't want to be seen with tears in my eyes. I have even used the simple trick that if you hold your head completely up, it becomes very difficult to cry. Huh, it doesn't work well—I know—I've tried it. When all this damn pain and hurt are inside, those two forces just push my head down, and I cry."

*   *   *

I slowly became more composed and apologized for the extent of my outbursts but still thanked her for listening. After a minute or so, she asked very quietly, "Do you think we could talk for just a few more minutes?"

I actually looked at her now; before this, my head was down. "Well, sure . . . I guess so," I responded wearily. My eyes were still blurry, and my breathing was still shallow.

"You probably recall that on the last time we met, I was concerned that you were feeling a bit down that day," she said. "We talked about some of the hot flashes and the lack of sleep and then how you fight the naps you know you should take, yet while you were weary, you seemed to be handling it. I brought up whether you might like to try one of the several medications available to, let's call it, to level out some of the ups and downs you are feeling." She looked at me in a way that implied a question.

I took a breath and said, "Oh yes, I do remember that." My voice was more of a moan than a clear response. "Ahhh, I guess I said that I would think about it, but I suppose I haven't." I gave a weak smile, raised my eyebrows a bit, and said, "Guess I'm not doing very well these days, am I?" I shrugged my shoulders. Tears started to well up in my eyes again. She smiled and nodded in agreement.

"Well, today I am a little more concerned about you," she explained. "When there is major stress on your body and it tends to get you down or even causes you to be discouraged, even a little depressed, it makes it all the harder for your body to heal itself. This is not a simple body-mind division."

She continued, "We know from clinical studies that when men have a heart attack and become depressed afterward, they have a much higher incidence of a second heart attack—and a more serious one—than those men who are not discouraged or depressed after the first one. In other words, it's important to keep a balance between the assaults on your body and the level of your moods. If your mood is way down, your body may not heal as quickly. Do you see what I'm saying?"

"Yes, I really do. I know I have been down in the dumps quite often." I paused and she waited. "I've even gotten sloppy about my appearance, my clothes. Ingrid mentioned my clothes and appearance one day, and I just shook my head and in a very negative tone said, 'Yes, but who cares?'

"'Well, I do,' she said firmly, and that took me back for a moment. I certainly wasn't being very pleasant."

"That's right, that's the idea; that's what I'm driving at," Dr. Shah said. "Why don't you try one of these two and see if that makes a difference for you; if it doesn't work, we can try another one."

"Well, what kind are they, and I guess the most important thing is . . . well, I get worried about the side effects." I was going to say something else, but I didn't even want to make a choice. So I just added, "Well, look, why don't you select the one you think is best for me, and I'll get it . . . ahh . . . oh, I can get it today since I have to be at the center at 12:30, and there's a drugstore nearby." I was not talking with much vigor or enthusiasm, but I was connected to this discussion. She handed me a prescription.

"So thanks for listening to me. I'm sorry for the way I behave, but this whole thing is just such a damn mess. I'll try this medicine."

We said goodbye; and before she left the room, I asked, "It's OK for me to sit here a little bit?"

"Absolutely." She nodded her approval. I sat quietly for a few more minutes.

*   *   *

As I left, I was very tired, but I was also relieved to have expressed so many volatile feelings. I can't remember how I got out of the reception area of office, but I am sure that I crept out so that no one would see me. I stopped in the men's room to wash my face; I wasn't sure whether I would look in the mirror. I took a quick look and said out loud to myself, "It's far worse than I thought." I washed my face several times as if I could wash away everything that happened. I couldn't. I sat in my car for about five minutes to let some energy return and to contemplate some of what had just occurred. I almost started condemning myself again for what I found myself to be, but I was too tired to do it.

I thought back to the things I had just said and realized that to talk out in such anger and disgust to someone else is a good way to hear yourself. I could sit all day and think those things, but it is only in the hearing that they have so much more meaning and emphasis. So much clarity. I learned about myself by simply hearing my own words. In these few moments sitting alone in my car, I could absorb their importance a little more.

Dr. Shah had done much for me, first, by having been a trusted physician as well as medical counselor for several years, by quickly and thoughtfully prescribing medications and planning tests when she saw possible problems emerging, by removing a number of skin cancers, and by listening to me and understanding me as a person.

But on this day especially, she helped me by being silent, by touching me, by listening, by not diverting me from some of my utterly outrageous comments, by not responding except to be present, to sit near me and look at me, to nod, and to listen to me express hate and more hate, primarily at myself.

Finally, Dr. Shah helped by handing me tissues and letting the tears come out without interruption, the tears that are an essential part of the healing process. She let me release all the venom within myself, and she never said the words that are so anathema to the crying patient: "Don't cry, everything will be all right." I knew at that time, and anyone crying as fully as I was knows that nothing, absolutely *nothing*, will ever be all right.

I would have to change, to learn that I was not deficient by crying and that dependence at this time is acceptable, that radiation hurts, that hormone therapy changes a person, that the combination of the two can be almost overwhelming, and it is acceptable to cry. Hadn't I even said that to some clients in the hospitals and social agencies in which I worked—that it was all right to cry about serious problems? I could say it with the "authority" of an employee in an organization to others, but I was totally, absolutely incapable of applying that basic principal to myself. How totally mixed up I had become! My feelings were totally divorced from my knowledge.

I had several short episodes of crying in following weeks, but never as much as this one. This day, today, however, was the turning point. My world did slowly, very slowly, get better, partly or perhaps primarily because I was willing to make the change to the most important thing I could do right now: become a patient.

As I sat in the car, I realized anew that crying "clears the air," and I would feel better when I reached the center. After all, I had my cry and probably wouldn't cry again today. Furthermore, I'd be glad to see Dr. Brooks for my regular appointment.

Whenever I am really angry or annoyed with myself, I call myself, either out loud or in my head, "Baily." As I started to drink some water and eat an energy bar, that's what I did this day; my comment was out loud, and it was not very forgiving: "Baily, you are really pathetic; get a grip on yourself. You're not growing old very gracefully, but maybe you could at the very least start trying."

I put a CD in the radio, started the car, and headed for the cancer center.

CHAPTER 12

One of the great benefits of a large team of practitioners is that there is a good choice of persons to talk with. A patient can have the opportunity to meet staff members who may not directly serve a patient. One person that I had not noticed was Elizabeth, an RN who sat at a station on the left side of the hallway as I entered. I confess that I was always looking to the right where the refreshments were available. She caught my eye a couple of times, and we began to talk.

I started to realize there are no secrets among staff about the needs of a given patient. That's the way it should be, and I learned that Elizabeth knew much about me.

Elizabeth's chair was on an elevated platform, and she often stepped off it. We talked standing up, so I thought of her as my "stand-up counselor." She wanted to know about my work in past years, and like Dr. Brooks, she wished to see me as more than a patient with a disease. Elizabeth supported me by recognizing the range of emotional assaults or reactions that patients have. She knew about my fight for control over what happened to me as well as my strong need for independence. One day she related her own recent experience of having inpatient care. She made it clear to me she gave everyone in the hospital a front-row experience of what hell is like. She appreciated what I was going through. I never wept when talking with Elizabeth, but I had tears in my eyes a number of times. We also laughed many times.

Another benefit of conversing with Elizabeth was this: off and on, she had to stop to relate briefly to other patients leaving or arriving. This meant that there were a number of breaks to think about what was just said, and that gave me the chance to think about the discussion, as well as introduce other subjects. This is in contrast to individual counseling where the discussion continues uninterrupted. I found her to have an encompassing but never-controlling warmth, and I was always glad to have her gentle counsel.

My spirits were generally down as I approached the last couple of weeks of radiation. Andrea and Sybil suggested I might want to talk with a social worker; I agreed. Cynthia, a licensed social worker, and I reviewed what I had experienced throughout the radiation treatment; once again I expressed my continuing anger over my dependence and my excessive tiredness and all the emotional ups and downs of treatment. A few of my expressions were similar to the ones I had shared with Dr. Shah, though not nearly so intense nor so long. But I shed more tears. I was very glad to discuss these again since pain and anger can never be released and resolved in a single meeting. Cynthia, as with Dr. Shah, helped me to review this period and acquire more perspective on it. She was a wise, clear-thinking person, and she had a profound understanding of the strong emotions and reactions evoked by cancer and its treatment. She knew the effects of cancer treatment on families and on individuals, whether it was a man or a woman who was being treated.

Cynthia also knew about life's transitions. She helped me to look at this treatment time as a significant part of life, just like other phases or major events that we all experience. Treatment for cancer is an intense experience for almost every patient, and that experience should be placed in to the ebb and flow of other meaningful life experiences, whether they are ones of joy and exhilaration or ones of sorrow and pain. Consequently, I now had to think through what I would return to after recovery. Change is often difficult, and the ending of certain events can be troubling, even those that may be painful. Saying goodbye is uncomfortable for many people, probably for most of us. I would need to say goodbye to this phase, to those who helped me through it, and to let it slip into the past. There was no need to "get it behind me," as a current saying goes, but to accept it as one more significant and meaningful, albeit upsetting, events of my life.

*   *   *

After my meetings with Cynthia and Elizabeth, I began to adapt a little better to the cancer center program, despite the fact that I was very tired from the accumulation of both treatments. Perhaps I was compliant, a bit more flexible and accepting of treatment *because* I was so tired. The other major factor that brought about this subtle, but real, change was my awareness of and pleasure in anticipating the end of radiation. It was rapidly approaching. I also began to think that I would probably succeed in completing the radiation treatment. I had not had such a vivid thought of completion until then. In the waning days of treatment, I could also view myself as a bit of a "veteran" of the system.

Each day had become predictable, consistent. Though the insides of my abdomen usually felt like popcorn exploding within a hot, tightly closed pan, life for me at the cancer center had become routine. I could foresee no extra radiation days, no setbacks, no surprises. I was reminded of the Broadway musical *My Fair Lady* with Rex Harrison singing, "I've grown accustomed to her face, it's second nature to me now." The lyrics in my mind became, "I've grown accustomed to this place, it's second nature to me now."

I thought again about the meeting with Dr. Shah and realized that I was more upset and angry at that time than I had ever been in my entire life. I wondered how I could ever have held so much anger within me. I scrutinized that event and asked myself whether I had released all my anger. Was there a residue of resentment still posed within me, ready to emerge at another time? Was there a reservoir of anger remaining, also demanding expression? I decided there probably was not. At the very least, I hoped there wasn't. It would be too much to handle again. At that late stage of radiation therapy, I thought I would be too tired to release it. I was depleted.

I was empty. Energy is required to express strong anger. Furthermore, I no longer felt desperate about my circumstances. My daily pattern at the cancer center was set, and I was fully engaged. I'd grown accustomed to *my* place, accustomed to *this* place.

Then my mind jumped to the 1960s when I worked in a children's hospital in Philadelphia. The small hospital was, in effect, the pediatric ward of Temple University Hospital. One of my roles there was in the child psychiatry division. Weekly meetings were held to discuss child patients and their parents. One day a psychiatrist referred to the continuing anger of one of his adult patients who had, in the analyst's view, "reached the bottom" of his very being. The analyst said that the only element left in the man was anger, anger, and more anger.

The clinical leader of the meeting said that if the only feeling left in the patient was anger, then the patient had not yet hit bottom. He said that "beneath all the anger, all the hate, all the strong negative feelings, beneath everything else, is love." That comment gave everyone something to ponder. The question for me, as a cancer patient, was whether I had hit bottom. How far down does a patient have to go? How much has to be released, to erase the pain, the exhaustion from physical changes and mood alterations, the distress, the fears, and, yes, the anger?

I did not view myself at that time as a loving person, but I did sense that perhaps I had hit bottom and removed all the anger in me that was related to the cancer treatment. My anger was intense, explosive, and short lived. It was not related to a lifelong expression of anger toward others nor hostility in personal relationships. Because I was cleansed—my anger and my violent feelings were released—I was able in the final days to begin to return to more typical behaviors. I became a little more balanced; I became . . . is the word "mellow?" No, I had not reached the plateau of a stable and tranquil mood, but I was able to look toward the completion of radiation therapy with a bit more self-control, more understanding, and a degree of self-assurance.

*   *   *

During the entire course of treatment, I had lunch six times with my son, Kenneth; daughter-in-law, Christine; and granddaughter, Isabelle. My son, Peter, made it a point to get home for several weekends. Those were all special times, and I appreciated their willingness to travel a good distance to meet me. The lunch meetings were certainly a way, as Dr. Brooks suggested, to find distractions from cancer treatment. I also rented a fair number of "talking books" to listen to in the car, plus some videos to watch in the evenings. I purposely selected humorous ones and then a couple of mysteries. When my daughter drove with me, we had lunch in restaurants that served the richer foods characteristic of decades past, thereby meeting the dietician's recommendations. On two nights, I stayed at a local B & B, thereby reducing travel time and energy and providing a change of scene.

Throughout all of the latter stage of my radiation treatment, my daughter often accompanied me to drive and provide a conversation partner. That helped considerably. I counted on her driving and did not resist her offers of help. When she drove, I could also catch a nap. Whenever I was driving, which was more than half the time, I was aware of my weariness; so I was extra careful in handling the car. I never had any type of problem on the road.

Weight gain continued slowly, partly due to my limited exercise and physical activity. For a few weeks toward the end of radiation, I did almost nothing but eat, sleep, rest, and go for treatment. The meeting with the dietician, the strong support of my oncologist and personal physician and the food preparation of my daughter assured the balance necessary to minimize some of the abdominal problems. Through the entire period of treatment, I gained nine pounds, 7 percent of my normal weight.

CHAPTER 13

In the final week of radiation treatment, I apparently had what might be called a complete conversion to doing all the right things during treatment, such as resting, taking naps, and maintaining the correct diet. A new large waiting area had just been completed during the last two weeks of my treatment, and it was relatively easy for patients to converse briefly with other patients as they sat at small tables and had refreshments.

I introduced myself and talked with a few other patients that I was rather sure were new. I had more than casual conversations with two men and their wives as the men began their radiation. If there was anything I stressed, it was the importance of "listening to their bodies" and resting when they had to. I related some of the physical struggles that I had, whether abdominal or sleep loss. I found I had to take naps, but I became mad because I had so little energy and could not get some important things done. Both men, and especially their wives, were pleased to hear what they might experience. I was careful to explain that their experiences might be quite different from mine. It was not possible to converse long with someone in the waiting room, since patients are called at any moment to leave the area for the radiation treatment.

My life then had come full circle. Years ago I had helped people to make various changes in their lives, primarily as it related to their children.

Then I had cancer treatment and could not adapt to changes for my own benefit. Slowly I came to terms with the rigors of treatment. Eight weeks later, having finally accepted these changes in myself, I could legitimately encourage others to adapt to treatment.

*   *   *

The last day was like a graduation ceremony, saying a quick or longer goodbye to so many staff. As bad as I felt from the beltline down, I was in high spirits. But there was a strong, sorrowful component, since I was saying goodbye to so many people who had cared for me. My last day was a Wednesday, and on the previous Monday, I handed out the following poem. Although addressed at that time to the cancer center staff, it certainly is addressed now to all those medical people who joined together to help me, as if in a single treatment service, albeit in separate buildings:

In Celebration of the Cancer Center
Radiation Oncology Staff

Acquiring a disease I'd hoped not to have,
        Given a diagnosis I'd rather not hear,
        With travel to a center I'd prefer to avoid, and
        Served by a staff I'd otherwise not meet,
        I became a prostate cancer patient—reluctantly.

Treatment begins, forty-three days to go

How could I foresee how well I would be served?
        Who set in place this complex treatment design?
        This blend of caring for the person with the vast technology
        of medicine,
        This mosaic of counsel for body, mind, spirit?
        From what source is the mission to heal so thorough?

So embedded in each person,
No matter the extent of education,
The professional identity, or
The role of each healer,
So that hope is held forth, and
Restoration is the prime vision?

Thirty-three days to go

You brought me into a circle of assurance
　　Where fears about life and death can emerge,
　　Where former life threats long thought settled emerge once again,
　　Where emotions, confused and bizarre reside,
　　Where birthdays, anniversaries may bring pain,
　　Where tears surge too fast from sources unknown,
　　And where feelings of elation bring sudden relief.

Twenty-three days to go

You enclosed me within a cloak of compassion
　　Where tears are released gently or swiftly,
　　Where knowledge of treatment gives new understanding,
　　Where time slows down, pauses, even stops,
　　Where quiet, contemplation both bring healing,
　　Where silence restores balance and composure,
　　So that tomorrow, indeed, becomes a new day.

Thirteen days to go

From your care and support I found strength
　　To tolerate the physical assaults of radiation,

To yield to alien hormones—restless, unruly,

To concede that sleep will rarely be restful,

To endure capricious abdominal disorder,

To accept finally the weariness that demands frequent rest,

And the tiredness that drains and makes me feel old.

Three days to go

You were the anchor when my spirits flagged low, and you laughed

    with me when my spirits soared.

You gave direction when I was off course.

You were steady when I faltered.

You were sure, reassuring when I could never be sure.

Your eyes were clear when I couldn't see through mine.

Your gaze was direct even as my gaze avoided yours, and

Your voice was gentle, when my only voice was tears.

One day to go

Finally, as if your abundant care were not enough,

    You became more than a friend to me,

    You included me in every way, with a smile, a word, a nod, a glance.

    You gave of yourselves in more ways than I could ever ask.

    Far more ways than I could ask.

Thank you.

May 1, 2003

About three weeks after starting radiation, I read the following poem, "Otherwise" by Jane Kenyon. It is, I believe, a profound message on the fragility of life. I included it with the above poem.

Otherwise

I got out of bed
on two strong legs.
It might have been
otherwise. I ate
cereal, sweet
milk, ripe, flawless
peach. It might
have been otherwise.
I took the dog uphill
to the birch wood.
All morning I did
the work I love.

At noon I lay down
with my mate. It might
have been otherwise.
We ate dinner together
at a table with silver
candlesticks. It might
have been otherwise.
We slept in a bed
in a room with painting
on the walls, and planned
another day
just like this day.
But one day, I know,
it will be otherwise.[17]

---

[17]   "Otherwise," copyright 2005 by the Estate of Jane Kenyon. Reprinted from
Collected Poems, with the permission of Graywolf Press, Saint Paul, Minnesota.

Richard A. Kauffman, an associate editor at the *Christian Century*, identifies Kenyon's poem as one of his favorites. He comments as follows:

> Preachers and poets have but two subjects, God and death. Everything else is just footnotes. But what about life? Indeed, we live most fully and poignantly in the awareness of our mortality, knowing that some day it will be otherwise. To remember every day that we will die, as St. Benedict advised, is not morbidity, it is being aware of and present with life. Jane Kenyon wrote this poem after her husband, the poet, Donald Hall, was diagnosed with cancer. She herself battled with leukemia, to which she succumbed just before her 48th birthday. God is not mentioned in this poem. Still, knowing that reality will someday be "otherwise" gives the ordinary routines of life—eating and working and walking in the woods and making love and sleeping—a luminous, almost revelatory quality. It shouldn't be otherwise.[18]

With a poem about the joys of life and the reality of death, by a poet who would face her own death from cancer, it comes as no surprise that I would read this poem many times over.

*   *   *

I did nothing but routine things at home the day after my last radiation treatment. The following day I went into the local bank. As I left the counter, I saw the assistant manager in her office, and she caught my eye and nodded her head to invite me into her office.

"I haven't seen you for quite a while; how are things going?" she asked as I sat down in one of the soft chairs.

---

18. Copyright 2003 *Christian Century,* Reprinted by permission from the March 22, 2003, issue of the *Christian Century*. Subscriptions: $49/yr. From PO Box 378, Mt. Morris, IL 61054.

"Oh, fine, but I've been a bit occupied with going for radiation treatment for let's see, the past nine weeks. I have prostate cancer. That's why I haven't been in here very often."

"Oh, I didn't know that," she said, with an obvious look of concern. "I'm sorry to hear you have cancer and for whatever you had to go through with treatment; but I have to say, you look fine, you look healthier." That comment surprised me.

"Oh, well, thank you," I responded, as graciously as I could.

"In fact," she added, "you look quite well, your face is fuller, and you've gained weight, haven't you?" She looked directly at me and leaned forward slightly, as if to emphasize this positive statement. "You look much better!" These were both firm, declarative statements; there was no equivocation here.

I have no knowledge whatsoever of what kind of look I had on my face when she said that, but I know what I felt inside. Shock is not too strong a word for what I felt. I simply could not believe this; there is no way that I could comprehend this comment. For about nine weeks, I had undergone an inward battle with myself, and with a lot of others, over weight gain, wondering how I would reduce it, hoping that someone, anyone, but especially a professional, would agree with me that it was no good to have this extra weight and that I would have to do something to get rid of it.

And here was one of my good friends saying that not only had I appeared to gain weight (that was true) but that indeed I looked better for having gained the weight. Furthermore, the additional weight made me look healthier. Maybe I did look better and healthier.

I stepped out the bank door and paused on the step, and while I was perplexed, I was also amused with what just happened. I was sure that I looked like a comic strip character appearing listless and confused, with the balloon or cloud above his head with nothing but question marks inside showing disbelief in the conversation just experienced.

As I drove home, I was tempted to write a letter to several of my friends at the cancer center telling them what had happened and accusing them of locating my friend at the bank and telling her what to say to me the next time I walked into the bank. This brief event had all the hallmarks of a conspiracy. I never wrote the letter but often wished I had, for they would have had one more laugh about me.

It was just two days after that meeting that I was driving on the road where one of my friends, Caroline, lives. She had helped me considerably following the death of my wife in 1996, and we had become good friends. Caroline is a very practical, realistic, and caring person. Jolly, full of energy, and a great conversationalist. I had not seen her for almost two months although we had talked on the phone a couple of times. Her car was in the driveway, and I decided to take a chance and stop in without notice. She was free, and I stepped into her kitchen; we hugged each other, and she said, "Let's have a cup of tea." I readily agreed. She was busy for a couple of minutes setting up the teapot, and we hadn't really looked closely at each other. We sat down, now facing each other, waiting for the water to boil.

She wanted to know how I was, how I was feeling; and when I paused for a moment to tell her, she gave me that extra look and asked, "Have you gained weight?" The question almost implied—how could you do this to me?

I had no way to deny this anymore. The objective appraisal of others that I looked heavier was just too much for me to avoid this new, compelling truth. The weight was obviously in my face, let alone around my waist.

"Yeah," I groaned, "I have, although I didn't necessarily want it. I wish I didn't have it, but . . . I got it."

"Well, on you it looks very good; you look much healthier . . . much."

"I appreciate that, Caroline, I do, I really do." This time I was not shocked, did not consider this still another part of the cancer center's conspiracy. I did not have a blank look on my face. There comes a time when you have to admit and accept who you are and what you look like. Tuesday, May 15, 2003, was that day for me.

We chatted about many things; I left Caroline's feeling like . . . well, like a different and healthier person.

CHAPTER 14

During the summer of 2003, my abdominal discomfort slowly diminished, and my interests returned to my usual activities. On October 15, 2003, I sent a letter to Dr. Donovan, my new urologist, who I would be seeing on November 5.

I referred to the fact that

The radiation therapy really exhausted me, and I am finally beginning to get back some energy. I have not slept well for a long time following the radiation therapy, and the hot flashes usually wake me two times a night, but I have had nights of four times, once of six times. I am just now beginning to sleep a bit better or at least fall back to sleep more rapidly after being up. Within the past ten days or so, I have been able to do the last of the activities I performed [on my woodlot] prior to all treatment: using my chain saw, hustling firewood, and now, climbing on the roof for chimney cleaning.

I now have osteoporosis [confirmed by a bone scan]. I am now increasing walking and bike riding and will also try weekly yoga and other physical exercises. I will also be taking medication to increase bone density.

All of the above is to request that I discontinue the hormone therapy as of my appointment with you. Otherwise, I was scheduled for a final month's injection. I ask for the discontinuation unless there is overriding research and medical evidence in [cancer treatment] literature that the one-year hormone therapy is essential to kill all cancer lesions or that there is strong evidence for or medical belief that a final month of this treatment is required for my particular recovery from PC.

The letter was clear in my request to have the hormone therapy discontinued, and that became a very brief disagreement. Dr. Donovan said it was essential not just for immediate treatment but for long-term survival from cancer. I was therefore given a three-month injection, not the one-month injection that I believed had been planned.

*   *   *

The literature on radiation states that bone weakening can be a result of treatment. However, I was a prime candidate for osteoporosis prior to treatment, since I am a white Anglo-Saxon male of small frame and weight. I probably had osteoporosis prior to treatment. I suspect the bone density may have decreased still more because of radiation; the test indicated that I had the worst deterioration of bone. In January 2004, I fell and broke my arm near the wrist. While it was a nasty fall, the break was small, and the surgeon stated that my bones did not appear brittle to him. This was the first time I ever had a bone break.

In the early months of 2004, I carried out a vigorous exercise regime, both indoors and out; and that helped me to gain more physical strength and to reduce my weight. I suffered no more breaks although I did have two falls equal to the one that broke my arm.

*   *   *

In the spring of 2004, I decided to purchase a heavy-duty new brush cutter for work on our woodlot. My other one was old and less reliable. After assembling the new one, which weighed over 250 pounds, I used it off and on for a couple of days and found it very difficult to handle. I began to realize that it was too heavy for me to drive. It was very difficult to turn, and I struggled with all my strength to steer it. I began to blame myself for a very bad decision and thought back to my concerns about the cancer treatment. I decided that my judgment was really poor. I called the company, and they said that no one had any difficulty in handling these machines. I told them my weight—almost 138—and they said that there were two women working at the plant who each weighed only 110 pounds, and they had no difficulty using machines that contained more horsepower than mine and, in fact, were heavier than mine. I felt very small, inadequate.

I talked to my son, Peter, who told me to do nothing, just wait and give myself time. *Time? Time—are you serious?* I thought to myself. *What difference would that make? That would only mean that I couldn't return the machine under the trial period.*

I never used it that summer, and when preparing to put it away for the season, I had to move it about three hundred feet to an old shed. I was suddenly surprised; it was easy to move. Then I began to move it all around, turning constantly. I was elated. The problem was not the machine. I was the problem. Sixteen months from the end of radiation treatment were required before I recovered my full strength. My son was right—wait.

After radiation was completed, I had periodic meetings with Dr. Brooks. During one of them, in 2004, I decided to ask him whether I had been "rushed" into treatment due to a rapid increase in the cancer. He looked back through the record and very casually said, "No, it was a normal procedure, nothing special."

This is proof that my sense of worry had been working overtime, and very convincing proof that I should have asked the question much sooner. I could have saved myself a great deal of concern.

CHAPTER 15

Bathroom mirrors are a very handy way to look at yourself and discuss something, since you are fairly close to the other person—or that image of yourself—and there is usually good light in the entire room. There is no way to hide in the shadows. I've felt that this setting improved the communication and enhanced the thinking process, since you can quickly see how the other person is responding. When the conversation is alone in your mind, there is a certain disadvantage, since the communication is only one way. How can you know how accurately you are responding to something since you—well, it is really very simple—you can't see yourself? You might know something in your head, but that other image may help to deny or confirm how you feel, or even give you new information about yourself.

Just as we can look at others and have a reasonable idea of how people are responding, we can look at ourselves and perhaps get the same impressions. There is an extra advantage here: we probably become a tiny bit more accurate in our perceptions by looking at ourselves, since we already know fairly well what we are feeling inside.

On Tuesday, November 9, 2004, I had such a conversation with myself. Washing up first thing in the morning, I brushed my right arm against my right chest and felt a little pain.

Huh, I thought to myself, *what's that?* I looked down at my chest but did not see anything unusual. Whatever it was, it was a different feeling.

In the mirror, I found a person who indeed had a puzzled demeanor. Then that look changed to one of a bit of a frown, thereby indicating more serious thinking, more puzzlement.

I then used my left hand to feel that same area and found that it was quite sensitive. Did I feel a thickening in the area?

Was that my fear, or was it my imagination?

"Gee, that little discomfort happened very quickly," I said to myself, and my mirror image said essentially the same thing.

I wonder what is going on in there, I mused. And now my mirror image told me that this could be more than something minor. I had never before felt such sensitivity in the nipple area or on either side of my chest. No insect had bitten me, nor had I scratched myself. I had not fallen; there was no external reason that I should have this slight pain.

Looking in the mirror, I found that my face looked a bit askew as I put my tongue between my teeth and had it protrude a bit to one side, pushing very slightly on the one cheek. I also noticed that my shoulders had shifted up just a bit, perhaps indicating a little concern about this change, or at least apparent change, in my body. Did this slight change in what we call body language mean that maybe I was more concerned than I let on to myself?

Then I looked in the mirror again, moving to the next step and thinking, *So what do I do now?*

My mirror response was to place both lips slightly inside the teeth and then with a little nodding of the head said, "I'll have to think more about this."

I continued washing, said goodbye to my friend in the mirror, and started my day, still thinking.

This is what I had to consider. Four days later, I would be on the train to Boston to spend one day with my son and daughter-in-law then fly to the Caribbean to meet my niece, also named Christine, for four days. Then my son, daughter-in-law, and granddaughter would fly down; and we would be together for almost a week. Then on the weekend of November 27, we were having a special birthday party for my daughter, Ingrid; and I did not want my prostate cancer nor this new sensitivity in my chest to be mentioned on vacation or at the gathering. My other son, Peter, would be there for the party, as well as my niece Christine and sister-in-law Esther; so we were looking forward to a pleasant family time. I decided to tell no one and would wait until later to notify my physician, Dr. Shah.

Three days later when I arrived at my son's house in Boston, I brushed my left breast with my arm and realized that my left nipple was just as sensitive as the right one. "Well"—I exhaled a deep breath and a soft moan—"that's just the way life goes, isn't it?" I said to myself.

I did not need my mirror this time to tell me how I felt.

Being away in a tropical place on vacation, I thought, *would enable me to forget about everything, especially possible growths.* It didn't. Walking around most of the time in only a bathing suit, I was more keenly aware of the sensitivity in my breasts. In addition, with no shirt or other garment on, I found I bumped or brushed myself on the chest more often. I still had a good vacation but wished a number of times that I could tell someone what was going on. Nevertheless, my personal promise of secrecy held.

*   *   *

The celebration for Ingrid went very well. On Monday morning, November 29, when all family members were back in place, I called Nancy, Dr. Shah's nurse.

"Hi, Nancy, this is Walter. I got a little bit of news, at least I hope it is just a little."

"What's going on?" she asked.

"Well, I seem to have some sensitivity in my right breast, right at the nipple area. And the left also feels the same way. So I don't know what's going on but thought I better call."

"OK, I'll let Dr. Shah know, and we'll get back to you." It didn't take long. Within an hour, Nancy called back, and I had an appointment with

Dr. Shah at 8:40 the next morning. I knew this was before regular hours, so I gathered that they saw it as important.

I arrived on time for the meeting.

"Good morning," we said to each other.

"Thanks for coming in extra early to see me," I said.

"Well, that's my job." She smiled.

"Yes, I know, but still, it's extra time from your family and other obligations."

She examined me thoroughly in the chest and abdominal area, checking glands under the arms while asking a number of questions, such as "When did this start?" "Ever have this problem before?" "Is there pain on the other side?" "Does this hurt here?" "Do you feel that?"

More questions followed. "How much soy are you drinking or consuming these days? I recall that you told me that you buy soy milk and also have used one of the soy high-protein powders," Dr. Shah observed.

"Right . . . for a while there, and that was a couple of months back, I was using the soy powder about four or five times a week. It was very useful in cereal and the high protein content made me feel better and I had more energy until about noon. More recently, I have been primarily using soy milk on cereal, often mixing it with 1 percent milk and then drinking some—" Before I could finish, she asked, "How much do you drink a day?" Dr. Shah's questions were coming very quickly now. She was obviously intent on getting more information and getting it fast.

"Not that much, I don't think, maybe four or five ounces at a time, maybe twice a day," I replied.

"How about tofu; do you eat that often—in meals, soups, stews?" she asked.

"The most is about once a week, sometimes not that often," I said.

"Well," she commented, "I don't think that is enough to cause any enlargement of breast tissue; if you had been using two to three times that much soy, then that would be different. You see, soy does have estrogen in it; and if there is substantial intake of soy, then that could contribute to both thickening in the mammary glands and even contributing to a lump. But we have to check this out further. I have already set up a first step, that is, a chest X-ray for you this morning. Then we'll see where to go from there."

"All right, thanks for setting this up so quickly, and I'll wait to hear from you," I said.

"Certainly, I'll call you." In this meeting, I learned more about Dr. Shah. She can become rapid, precise, and intense during an examination, changing according to patient physical or emotional needs. I already knew that she can be as gentle as a barely audible sigh.

Dr. Shah contacted me by phone a couple of days later to say that the chest X-ray had been inconclusive, and an ultrasound for both breasts was set up for December 6 in the late morning. I had had an ultrasound before and believed this would be simple. It was, but I did not know that much more than an ultrasound would be required.

CHAPTER 16

My appointment for an ultrasound of both breasts was in the morning of December 6, 2004, at the hospital. The exam was completed, and I was in a chair in the hallway, awaiting approval to leave after the pictures were assessed for clarity. The nurse at the desk called and told me that the ultrasound examination was inconclusive. The radiologist said it was important to do mammograms today, right now, or right after lunch. I was surprised by this rather immediate request, and I agreed to return at 1:00 p.m.

Up to this time, I had been concerned about what was going on in my chest. My worry genes were alert but in normal operating mode. But when the word "mammogram" was used, this sounded more serious, and my worry gene team was called into emergency session. Just when I thought I was on a comfortable downhill slope, I was suddenly facing rugged terrain. I thought I could handle thoughts of cancer in the morning and evening, but now I wondered if I would have formidable worries about cancer in the middle of the night. That's when your worst fears emerge.

*　　*　　*

Mammograms are an essential tool for both the identification of benign or cancerous growths in female breasts, for planning the surgical removal of growths, the use of radiation beam therapy and other therapies in treating growths. They are also used for continued evaluation during and following a treatment regime.

Males have the same type of breast tissue as females. Young boys and girls up until puberty have the same tissue that consists of tubular passages located under and around the nipple. Following puberty, a girl's ovary produces female hormones, causing breast ducts to grow, milk glands to form at the ends of ducts, and fatty and connective tissue to increase. In contrast, the male hormones prevent any further growth of breast tissue. As with any cells in the body, a man's breast duct cells can have cancerous changes. It is likely that women have more breast cancer than men because their cells are continually exposed to the growth-promoting effects of female hormones.

Breast cancer occurs in males as well as females, but the national rate of male cancers is very low: one male for every one hundred females. This low incidence probably contributes to the low level of public awareness of the problem. The National Cancer Institute estimates that 1,690 men in the United States would get cancer of the breast in 2005, and 460 men would die from the same disease. Male breast cancer predominates in the age group of sixty to seventy.

The discovery of growths almost immediately raises life-threatening fears for women, even though approximately 80 percent of growths discovered for the first time are benign. Nor are growths in a man less threatening. I did not anticipate that I would be getting mammograms when I first discussed this apparent lump in my right breast with Dr. Shah. I may have been in total denial about the possibility of breast cancer, in spite of the fact that I had just been through prostate cancer.

A reasonable question I should have considered was whether there had been some spread from the prostate to the breast, even though I knew that any metastasis almost always occurs closer to the original site. It is most likely to go into the bones in the pelvic area. For some reason, I was rather casual about believing that the cancer had spread and was now located in my breast. Had I forgotten already that I previously denied a serious disease? I may have had minimum concern at this time because my PSA scores over a two-year period had been at zero—or 0.003. As my urologist said at a previous time, "That's not even measurable."

* * *

I arrived at the radiology area a few minutes before 1:00 p.m. As I sat in the hall and waited for the technician, I thought to myself, *Well, here we go again, another rush to treatment.* That sounds like a negative, or at the very least a cavalier attitude; it really wasn't. It was partly the excitement of becoming a part of the "chase" as it were, to be a small part of the effort to discover whether there is a lump and what to do about it. I was glad that Dr. Shah had moved so quickly, since I had waited so long to inform her, and I was beginning to wonder what kind of a problem I might have. Instead of fear, I thought that it would be certainly unusual, perhaps almost strange to have mammograms when I was so slim. Might it even be amusing to try to get clear mammograms on me?

The closer I got to the exam, the more I began to have some concern. However, I became so involved in this entire process of trying to get a good mammogram that I lost most of my worry about cancer. In a small way, I was now a partner in the effort to get vital information.

The technician, who is a registered technologist in radiography (RTR) met me on time in the hall, introduced herself by name, Janet, and invited me back to the examining room. I didn't know what to expect, but I certainly thought the room would be larger than it was; I was accustomed to the larger rooms where chest and other full body exams are taken.

This room was about twelve feet by fifteen feet with one corner completely enclosed for processing films. A small desk was in one corner with a lead-reinforced thick glass in front of it. This area was for the technician to move behind to operate controls and to remain there when mammograms were taken.

The mammography machine, standing in one corner, was basically a rounded post that holds a boxlike X-ray unit. The latter contains a grid at the bottom that holds a film cassette, a Plexiglas paddle in the middle that moves up and down, called a platform, and a larger enclosed plate at the top that sends the X-ray beam. The bottom plate is positioned a bit below chest height.

The entire box arrangement can be raised or lowered as well as placed in a horizontal or vertical position. Therefore, the entire unit can be adapted to the height and size of any person. In addition, the Plexiglas unit or paddle can be raised or lowered so the breast can be gently held in place to minimize or prevent movement when the mammogram is taken.

The technician operates, with her feet, four levers on the floor to adapt this assembly to each person. In setting up the patient for the X-ray, the RTR must gently push and move, or instruct the patient, to a precise place within the assembly.

When Janet asked me to remove my undershirt, stand close, and face the lower plate, I watched briefly and could see the logic of this design for mammograms on females. I was not feeling so sure about its usefulness for a man, and a slim one at that. We started with the entire assembly in its natural upright position.

I can't say whether she pushed me into the plate or placed me close to it, but there was no doubt that I was beginning to have a close connection with that part of the box. I watched with fascination as she moved her feet over the several foot levers to get this box to conform to my torso—or vice versa. Janet was finding it difficult to place me in a position that had my breast out far enough to get a picture, since I really didn't have any breast.

Since the entire unit cannot be positioned at an angle from the rounded, vertical post (the entire arrangement rotates on a single coupling), the only position I had to take was to place my feet forward under the unit. Otherwise, I would be leaning over the lower plate or grid, and that would have given a picture of a few ribs, and not much more. But in placing my feet under the plate, I was leaning far back on my heels and about to fall backward.

"I'm going to fall over, Janet," I announced.

"No, you won't," she said. "Hold it a second. Don't breathe."

"I can't stand up," I said. I moved backward, wondering if I would trip.

"All right, let's do this again," Janet said. She set me up with the same arrangement.

"I'm still going to fall."

"Don't," she told me. She paused a moment. "Just move your heels back, and you won't fall."

I tried and I was still going to fall and I told her that. Then I saw directly in front of me a small upright handle-type bar at the side of the assembly. I grabbed it with my right hand just as she was about to go to the desk and take the photo.

"Can I hold on to this handle?" I asked.

"No," was Janet's firm response, "I'll get nothing but muscle; I've got to have tissue, not muscle."

She came back from her safe location behind the glass. She arrived quickly since it is only about three or four steps from the desk to the machine. Janet was neatly dressed and a little taller than I am. She could move very quickly from one place to another, taking long strides in this very small area. The fact that she was so obviously motivated to get completed films made me more willing to cooperate with her as best I could.

"All right," she announced, "let's do this again. We'll get it." I was quickly realizing that this technician knew exactly what she was doing. It was becoming obvious to me that she probably had a large set of skills and positions available to match any torso or body size, protrusion, or shape, including that of a man, even with a torso like mine.

Janet said to me, "OK, now let's get you back to the same position; now put your head back a bit, your chest a little more forward and get your feet up there, and put your heels—that's right—get your heels closer there. Now can you hold that?"

"I'll try, but I'm still off balance," I said. "Tell you what, let me hold that handle bar for a second, then I'll let go just as you tell me you're going to click, and maybe that'll do it."

"OK, ready, don't breathe." *Click.*

I almost fell over backward.

"Let's see what this looks like," Janet said. She went behind the door and came out in about two minutes. "No good."

"Oh, too bad." My voice trailed off as I shared her disappointment.

"All right, lean into it again," she stated. "We'll get you into a slightly different position." I knew that Janet was slightly heavier than I am, slightly taller, and an experienced professional; now I was learning that she was physically strong. She pushed and adjusted, moved and removed, positioned and repositioned me several times to get me in the precise location she wanted. But as far as I could tell, it was the about the same position as before, and I might fall again.

"All set?" she inquired. She was still pressing me into the plate.

"Yeah, but I'm still going to fall over."

"Try not to. I have to go behind the lead barrier, so I can't push you into the machine. Now hold your breath." She was fast; the click sounded before I lost balance.

She almost ripped the film out of its cartridge and took it into the processing room. A minute later, she emerged.

"Nothing," Janet said. I could almost feel that the mood in the room had become somber.

She tried again with the same result.

She decided to show me the evidence so far of what I now considered our joint effort to get a clear photo. She let me know that she had only seen four men in the past four months, and it is sometimes quite difficult to get good mammograms on men.

She held up a film that was basically a black, thick line at the bottom, with a wisp of a white streak above the black. Above that was nothing but dark gray emptiness. I even thought to myself, *Rather depressing.*

Any thought of depression or despair quickly passed, and Janet became fully engaged in completing this task. We did three more shots, and they all produced just about the same amount of blackness. A biblical phrase came to me from the first chapter of Genesis: "The earth was without form and void."

"All right, let's try this again, except with a little difference," she announced. My left side was pushed against the lower grid, and the paddle was then lowered as she touched, faster than any tap dancer I had ever seen, the small levers on the floor. As I watched and felt the part going down, I had beginning worries of an out-of-control vise about to crush the little bit of flesh that I had on my chest. Although I had total confidence in Janet up to this point, I wondered what would happen if she missed one of the levers or she tripped and the two parts would crush, well, simply crush the skin on my chest. I should not have worried. Janet, as I began to find out, was an expert. I was in a good position on the platform, and she clicked the shot.

The same routine followed once more with no results. All was silent.

Then I heard a different type of breathing, the type of firm, well-measured breathing that occurs when one is deciding what to do or when something has to be done, has to be done right and has to be done now. With a hint of accusation, but one that also carried both compassion for me and determination for what the next step would be, she said, "You're *nothing* but skin and muscle! I have to have tissue. I *have* to have *tissue!*"

I was briefly startled by this declaration. I started to feel apologetic, almost troubled that I did not have the major ingredient that she needed to get a good photo—tissue. The word "useless" crept into my mind. I was hanging on to one of the forbidden handles waiting for her next announcement of what was going to happen. It came promptly.

"All right," she announced, "we're going to do a cleavage!"

I was momentarily frozen in place. Then I looked at her sideways, disbelief on my face, hoping I could find somewhere in her expression that she was not really serious, that all of this was a joke, and I could go home soon. I turned farther to my right, looked directly at her, and asked, "Cleavage?" My mouth was held partly open, wanting to say more; but no more words could come out, no matter how I tried.

"Cleavage," she answered firmly, as if to say, "Don't question my decision!"

"You're kidding." My question was swept aside by her rapid response.

"Cleavage!"

Her statement was a conclusion, not a proposal. It was not open for discussion. It was at this moment that I saw another part of Janet. Her eyes.

All of her conviction, all of her determination about this specific job was fully contained in her eyes. I decided to ask no questions. I would obey what she said. This indeed was a person on a mission. It was fully embodied in her clear, dark eyes.

As she moved toward me, I backed up a little and realized that I had been holding on to the handle, this time for emotional support, not for physical balance.

Back to the plate again, but this time a little differently. Both sides of me under that damn upper moving part that was beginning to remind me of a crushing machine in an automobile graveyard. This was not going to be one side, but both sides of me under threat of extinction. From behind, she pushed and repositioned me so that my chest was over the lower part of the platform, and my legs were slightly under the unit. I did my best to hold that position, and she flipped the switch.

Result? Zero.

Janet was not fazed. She described another technician, who recently came to the hospital and had X-rayed more people in six months than most lab technicians do in a year. Janet went out, and a few minutes later they both came in. The new one, named Louise, arrived with a certain fierceness in her eye that was both reassuring and daunting. I figured that the odds were now three to one: the vice grip machine and two determined RTRs all lined up against me. Then I realized this was not against me; it was against a portion of my torso that refused to yield its secrets to anyone, especially to this machine.

We went through the same steps except for the cleavage picture. I have never been pushed, shoved, rearranged, held, squeezed, instructed, directed, and repositioned in such a short time than on this day. I was permitted on one shot to hold on to the forbidden handrail. They were so determined to get the photos that on two of the shots Louise stood behind me, pushing firmly against both sides of my back, forcing me against the machine while the mammograms were taken. They assured me that the dosage was very low in this machine, so Louise would not be harmed. *Hey,* I thought to myself, *what about me? I'm the one that's been getting all the radiation!* I counted as best I could, and a total of twelve or fourteen mammograms were taken. I did not know whether any of them obtained clear shots of tissue.

We called it a day, and I turned and thanked both of them a couple of times for their extra effort. They both agreed they were glad to do this and wished me well.

Louise left promptly; and I said to Janet, "Well, this was really quite a day; there's nothing funny about taking mammograms and the worry that women will have about growths and cancer, but for a skinny guy like me, I have to say it was unusual and maybe a bit amusing. If I would ever try to write something about all my experiences with prostate cancer, this would certainly be, at least for me, one of the funnier parts."

Just as I found her to be creative and skilled in operating a complex machine, to have firm and clear ways to acquire clear mammograms, and finally to make rapid decisions without equivocating, I finally recognized her great pride in and commitment to her profession. I tried to convey my respect for the difficulties she must face with many patients, especially when they are extremely upset about the prospect of breast cancer. It takes patience and compassion to serve patients who are worried, anxious, and fearful. Her job required far more than simply taking mammograms.

We walked down the hall next to each other quietly. Janet asked me to wait in a small waiting room. My daughter joined me a few minutes later, then Janet returned, and I was glad to introduce each to the other. She let me know that the radiologist had completed review of the mammograms; we said goodbye. She left and was immediately taking another patient for mammograms. I wondered how tired she was from serving a male patient, and I was certainly a difficult one on which to obtain a satisfactory mammogram. When we reached the car, Ingrid sensed that I was tired, and she drove. I thought of Janet still working in her lab. The mammograms were started at 1:05 p.m.; we left there at 3:15.

*   *   *

As we headed home, I began to rest from what was, certainly for me, a whirlwind of activity. Janet had been quiet as we first walked down a long hall together. Medical personnel often make light chatter about the weather, if I live in town, but Janet did not. Maybe she was preoccupied with other things, but perhaps not. What might she have been thinking when she saw that her patient was a small man, probably light of weight, and certainly old? After all, she did know my birth date. Would she have said to herself, *This will not be easy since he may be thin, but I'll do what I can?*

Then when I took off my top shirt and she saw that I was really thin, she may have thought, *This is going to be tougher than I thought.*

Then when I took off my undershirt and she saw my skin, slightly drawn, even withered now from older age, then saw my nonmuscular appearance, especially in my arms—somewhat depleted from the effects of radiation, hormone therapy, and insufficient exercise during winter—and finally saw thin skin covering a small rib cage, did she think, *Does somebody really expect me to get mammograms on this patient?*

Maybe she had those thoughts, but if she did, I firmly believe they were only fleeting. Janet, in my estimation, used every strategy from her knowledge of anatomy, both male and female, and from her repertoire of skills with this large inanimate machine to make it perform. The more I thought back to what she did, and perhaps what she did not do because it was not suitable for my situation, the more I realized that I had been in the presence of a medically skilled professional totally devoted to choosing and adapting whatever materials and equipment must be manipulated to acquire essential data on which other staff will treat a patient. Janet was talented, creative, committed, and energetic. Perhaps she was thinking to herself, *This man probably has a growth in his breast somewhere and maybe another one on the other side. He's already had prostate cancer, and maybe this will be breast cancer. I'll do whatever I can to try to get the needed data so that he can be successfully treated.*

I did not learn whether the additional mammograms took or not, but I received a letter a few days later that I was being referred to another hospital for another series of mammograms and for examination by a surgeon. Dr. Shah met with me before that and explained that growths were evident from Janet's mammograms. That was the basis for the referral to the other hospital. When the surgeon examined me on December 14, 2004, he said clearly that there were growths present in both sides even before the new mammograms were taken. He also said there was no apparent metastasis into the glands under my arms and neck.

At the other hospital, eight more mammograms were taken, and it was a similar process. The technicians never said it; but I'm convinced, based on the way they had to repeat mammograms, that they also had some thick black lines. But after meeting Janet, this current exam for me seemed more formal, more routine. Stand here, lean this way, that way, don't breathe, *click*. There were two technicians; both were courteous and thoughtful, but there was minimum communication between us. They said nothing about the clarity of the mammograms.

CHAPTER 17

Surgical removal of the two growths—both benign—was on January 4, 2005. My next appointment with Dr. Donovan, the urologist, was on January 19. I wanted to make sure that I had a letter in the urologist's hands prior to meeting with him so that I could understand whether I might have more lumps develop and especially what might be done about the continuing hot flashes. I had begun to define them as "glows." They certainly compared in no way to some of the real wildfires that swept through my body when I was under the full force of the hormone therapy.

My two-page letter, dated January 10, 2005, was a quick summary of my experience with the hormones and the fact that they were continuing even though my last injection was almost fourteen months ago. It was obvious that I had concern about the breast lumps and continuing hot flashes or I would not have used two full pages to review my concerns. A few of the sentences follow:

> Is there any likelihood that there might be more growths in breast tissue in the future? I ask this because you had mentioned that it was rare for there to be breast sensitivity this far away from the use of (hormone therapy).

You did mention that there is a medication that can compensate for the flashes; is that something to consider? I am always reluctant to take medication if I can avoid it and more than willing to do other things to avoid a medication . . .

If the side effects are worse than the flashes, then that has to be taken into account.

Could it be that my hormone system has been more than temporarily changed so that I need some medication to reverse whatever new hormone pattern has been put into place? Is that conceivable? Can a new hormone pattern be established that might be irrevocable? Possible?

I continue to wonder why the Lupron medication is not calibrated for body weight or perhaps for testosterone levels, although I know those levels vary periodically. I remain puzzled that I as a 130-pound man would receive the same quantity as a 260-pound man.

On the day of my appointment, Carl, his nurse, stopped in to see me first. I explained what had happened recently. He was surprised about the growths, and I assured him that I seemed to be fully recovered and hoped that this was the last of it.

Dr. Donovan walked in a couple of minutes later with the bounce of a man who absolutely enjoys his work and likes to meet with patients. He immediately announced that he had gotten my letter. He said there would be no more lumps, absolutely not. I was surprised, but what more could I ask?

He also reported with pleasure that once again my PSA was 0, or so low that no measurement could be taken. I recalled that my second one taken six months after the beginning of the Lupron injections was 0.003, again not even measurable. In contrast to my previous appointment, he wanted to give me a DRE to make sure that the gland was smooth, having no irregularities that could be indicative of cancer. I leaned over and had to breathe a little differently because of the sudden pressure in the anal area.

As I dressed, we began to talk about the continuing hot flashes, and he said they would absolutely stop. He then explained that the one clear solution to the flashes is radiation on both breasts. A number of men have had this. Not many units of radiation would be necessary, but the hormone apparently can reside in the breasts, and the radiation treatments would remove the vast majority of it.

He added, "But of course there would be side effects." He had pencil and pad in hand and asked whether he wanted me to sign up.

I said, "Let's wait. I want to think about it and want to talk with my children about it."

"Sure?"

"Yes," I said. "Frankly, I'd rather continue with the flashes I have now than to take on more radiation and then have to deal with that. Radiation really depletes me."

We then talked briefly about my health other than with the cancer. I said, "I am truly fortunate with my health; I have no serious problem with which to contend. While I have arthritis, it is not the debilitating kind; then I have osteoporosis. I have a bit of bad cholesterol that should be reduced by a different diet, and I'm currently taking a low dose of Lipitor. Then I take an aspirin and a calcium pill."

He said to me several times, with a big smile, "Olive oil, olive oil, olive oil," to which I totally agreed. I didn't tell him that our family has consumed enough olive oil to affect the price on the world market. I mentioned a couple of other aspects of my favorable health; and he smiled, almost laughed as he said, "You look very healthy."

I thanked him, and we shook hands.

He grabbed the case record and said, "Come on back with me to the secretary."

I followed; and as he handed her the chart to prepare for the next appointment in six months, he turned to me with a bright radiance and said, "The last time you were here I thought this, and today I think it again—the saying is 'What a wonderful life!' You have a great life."

I was taken aback by his comment; and I quickly said, "Thanks," but only a split second before his secretary said, "I think the same thing."

I left there with a heightened sense of well-being.

*　　*　　*

The following weekend, I slowly became aware that my hot flashes did not seem as strong as before. How does one measure that? There were no objective criteria I could use, but I sensed that something was changing. Then I began to make careful notes of when they occurred and whether they seemed to arrive for reasons unrelated to anything I might be doing or eating. I was surprised, pleased, but then I began to wonder if I were engaged in wishful thinking.

On January 23, 2005, a Sunday, I really believed they had diminished in heat and frequency. But the real test would come during the night when they awaken me. The night ones were much less intense—no more throwing off the covers and almost ripping my pajama top off and throwing it as far away as I could, saying, "Dammit, get away from me." Then I had my first night without a hot flash. "I hope every last one of you dies," I said aloud, as if they could hear me, since I almost believed they were live demons. On February 2, 2005, I sent the following letter to Dr. Donovan:

> I hesitate to write this letter for fear that what I am about to tell you will change. We met on January 19th and the following weekend, especially on Sunday the 23rd, I sensed that I was not having the usual number of hot flashes, that they had probably dropped to two or three a day. Then the next night I slept through without a single hot flash. During the next few days I was then more attentive to the presence (or absence) of them, and finally it became clear that they were diminishing, down to two, then one, then for four nights in a row, nothing.
>
> As of today I am (dare I say this?) almost positive they are gone. Let's not talk about this, don't tell anyone; they might

come back and haunt me. Some things have a life of their own, you know.

To what can this remarkable disappearance be attributed? Do you really have a magic wand? The Magic Touch that we all want? Well whatever this is, it calls for some kind of a celebration. Thanks; you were right, you told me they would go away, but did you really believe they would depart as if you commanded it?

I will tell others of your remarkable talents. Hello to Carl.

Enjoy Spring.

It takes no special awareness to notice how different this letter was from most of the others. I had suddenly been released from the annoyance, the drag on my life, the interference of heat surges at any time of day or night. I was now freed to have a consistent body temperature. No wonder that my letter was so spirited.

Then on the night of February 7, I slept through the night. That was the third night that I could recall that I slept all the way through. I couldn't think of anything I did the day before to warrant this change, except that I retired about an hour and a half later. It is sheer joy to get up in the morning and realize that you have not been awakened. It makes it possible to bounce out of bed and into the day. I knew, or certainly understood, that the hormones would really leave, and I was told that the flashes would cease about three to four months after the last injection. Mine lasted more than one year beyond the expected time.

CHAPTER 18

It was almost two and a half years from the day I learned I had cancer to the end of the hot flashes. When I started, I thought the process would be over in about seven months. The typical time for this process is about fifteen months.

I was fortunate in the types of treatment received and the many persons who served me. In spite of internal turmoil, loss of muscle volume and strength, emotional ups and downs, weariness and anger, I have recovered. My weight is back to normal, my physical strength has essentially returned, and my general health is good. I am back to my pretreatment diet. The radiation probably increased or perhaps guaranteed the loss of bone strength, but I may have had osteoporosis before the radiation. I sleep well and get up only once at night. My last two PSA tests were three tenths (0.3). That number is expected to increase slowly to a low whole number. I will be followed by Dr. Donovan, the urologist, for another three years, and subsequently by Dr. Shah, my family physician.

What did I learn about this disease and my response to it? When I first heard the word "cancer," I treated it lightly, pretended—even said to others—that it was a "garden-variety" illness. Treatment would be quietly completed in several months. I deceived myself by believing that prostate cancer, unlike other cancers, was not as lethal, not as debilitating. I was forced, via an alarming nightmare, to recognize that I had little control over what was happening; and I could be seriously impaired or die. What I had to do was cooperate completely with the treatment and its consequences. To do otherwise was folly. I submitted myself, after much resistance, to become a patient and only a patient.

I could blame the cancer and the consequences of treatment for some of my problems. However, I brought the seeds of problems with me—the type of work I had in the past, the death of my wife and whether I could have prevented that; how some past and current events, especially those full of emotion, can pile up all at once and cause distress; how I treated cancer as if it were a sore throat; and how I hated dependency. What person does not have unresolved problems or events from the past? As I learned more about treatment and accepted its consequences, my fears and my resistance slowly subsided, and my behavior changed.

The one question that continued to interest me was why the periodic hormone injections that I received to control testosterone were not calibrated according to body weight. After I had fully completed the treatment program, I had the chance to talk with another urologist, not my own, about this subject. He recognized the validity of the question and said the answer was probably rather simple: no study has yet been conducted to determine what benefits, or lack of them, relate to the quantity of leuprolide injected.

A short time after that, I was perusing another medical Web site[19] and found that the same medication I received was given to boys who had developed premature adult male characteristics. That problem can be diminished or corrected by using hormone therapy, and the quantity of the medication *is adjusted according to body weight.* I finally found a partial answer to my question.

I hope research will be conducted on this question to assess whether the quantity of the medication does or does not affect its effectiveness in treating prostate cancer and whether varying amounts would minimize the

---

[19.]   www.MedlinePlus.com, The National Library of Medicine and the National Institutes of Health.

well-known side effects of androgen deprivation therapy. I am aware that this question may not be vital to cancer treatment, but it may be one more element in the increasingly large number of strategies and choices available for types, timing, and sequencing of treatment.

My observation here is not a criticism as much as a recognition that research is constantly ongoing and that not everything can be known as quickly as either patients, medical practitioners, or researchers would prefer. It is also a reminder that both patients and physicians can never know all there is to know prior to engaging in a treatment regime. Much is known, and I, for one, have been very grateful for the ways in which that knowledge and experience were used to help me.

The possibility of cancer recurrence will be present as long as I live. If the disease should return, I will be a different person—very different. I'll know what to expect and know how to adapt to it.

CHAPTER 19

After reviewing this record of my experience with cancer treatment, some might wonder about my emotional or physical strength. I looked extensively for data on the percent of men who experienced problems related to treatment. There are small studies on various side effects but no comprehensive research on patient characteristics and side effects. How many men weep, how many men are erratic, and how many men are totally depleted at any time during treatment? I certainly questioned whether I was strong a number of times.[20] But consider the following small event:

---

[20]. The range and intensity of emotional problems that both men and women face with cancer are presented very clearly by Roger Granet, MD, *Surviving Cancer Emotionally: Learning How to Heal,* John Wiley, 2001. The author, a psychiatrist, presents many case illustrations of the very serious problems that some patients face during treatment, with a very few to the point of requiring inpatient psychiatric care. Persons have a wide range of serious reactions relating to fears of death, changed relationships with loved ones, guilt over failure to obtain treatment, identification with relatives who died from cancer, even the wish to die—in effect committing suicide by delaying treatment or refusing treatment. Because many persons face a variety of problems does not mean everyone will.

A year or so before cancer treatment, I needed a new chain saw. My daughter and I went to a shop that carries all equipment for loggers and timber operators. The proprietor is known to be a tough man, and he had been a logger for years. We were looking at some of the saws, and he walked over. He was twice my size. I told him I wanted to get a new saw; and I understood the Husqvarna, made in Sweden, was a good one.

With no hesitation, he said, "This is the only one for you." That was a directive, not an idle comment. He picked up the saw with one hand as if it were a small kitchen utensil and showed it to me.

"Oh," I replied as I paused for a moment. "But why this one?"

He looked down at me and said, "Because you're getting *old*, that's why. In a couple of years, you probably won't even be able to pick this machine up, let alone start it!" I wondered how to respond to a comment like that.

Putting on my best smile, I said, "Gee, I guess the next time I want to be insulted I'll come over here." And without giving him a split second to reply, I asked in a very friendly way, "So what is there about this one? Must be a good reason."

"See this button here? It's a decompression device so that when you pull the cord, you're not pulling against the force of the engine compression, so it's much easier to start. It's excellent for older men." There was that word "old" again.

I picked up the saw, and it had a good feel to it. It also had excellent balance. My daughter and I agreed it was a good idea; I bought the saw.

More than two weeks later, I called him on the phone and stated that I didn't think the button was working. It still seemed quite hard to pull the starting cord.

"What are you doing?" That wasn't a question. As before, it was a directive.

I thought a second and said, "I pull the button out and then start pulling the cord."

"You pull it *out?*" he growled with disbelief.

"Yeah," I said softly.

There was a split second pause, and he declared firmly, "You don't pull it *out*, you push it *in*." I was silent.

He then stated slowly and clearly, with an inflection and question at the end, "Do you mean to tell me you've been using that saw for two weeks without using the decompression button?"

"Uhh, yes."

After a one-second silence, I heard the following carefully and slowly articulated statement: "Man, you *are* one hell of a lot tougher than I thought you were."

APPENDIX

For those men who will need and seek treatment for prostate cancer (PC), the types and range of treatment will be quite different from that provided in 2003 and 2004. The quality and extent of services may partially depend on where a person lives, the access to cancer services, and the patient's acceptance of the services offered. Some patients may choose to, or find that they must, live elsewhere to obtain needed services.

The good news is that improvements are being made in the types of treatments, the effectiveness of complex equipment, the efficacy of new medications, the reduced invasiveness of procedures, and the management or reduction of serious side effects. Research and clinical trials are underway for the reduction of treatment times, as well as the combinations of treatments available. However, specific types or combinations of treatment and equipment, including the medical specialists to operate them, will not be available in every community, just as they are not available everywhere today.

The following is a brief review of some emerging treatments and cancer treating equipment, coordination of treatment, when additional treatment should be employed, the management of side effects, and what posttreatment services should be offered. While almost all content in this chapter is derived from the Internet (reports are from around the world), the original sources are from professional journals, official press releases from medical centers, and research organizations. When articles from these several sources have been written or condensed by nonmedical writers,[21] then content may not be accurate nor emphasize the major thrust of the investigators.

---

21. Readers should also note that this writer is a nonmedical person.

Research studies with control groups and large numbers of subjects always carry more weight than treatments in research projects without control groups, without double blind studies, those called preliminary investigations, or those named phase-one studies. Studies may also apply to only one class of patients, such as those who have early, moderate, or advanced stages of cancer. Age and general health status may also limit the application of the findings to all patient groups. Some treatment medications may apply primarily to patients who have a recurrence of prostate cancer. Some studies are confined to only one institution while others will apply to a large group of patients from many cancer centers. Consequently, a patient should talk with one or more cancer specialists before choosing a course of treatment. It is unwise to select treatment based on what a given study may conclude.

In spite of the above reservations, this material gives a fair sample of some of the new forms of treatment devices, procedures, medications, intensity of treatment, and reviews of existing practices. This section is only intended to present changes and advancements taking place recently, not a full description of all services and treatments for prostate cancer. Some of these findings contradict each other. That is not surprising; differences may relate to the characteristics of the investigation, the number and size of the studied population, the treatments offered, and other features. Contradictions are actually a benefit, since they challenge researchers to refine their studies so that the probable causes of cancer and the reliability and effectiveness of treatment can be more firmly established.

Finally, the information here does not include anything related to the prevention and treatment of other forms of cancer or to basic cancer research. The latter research and studies about other types of cancer may well have application to prostate cancer. An example of this is the finding that stem cells may also be cancerous. This is in contrast to our common knowledge that stem cells are healthy and contribute to the control of disease and removal of disabilities. While most of the cells in a tumor contain diseased cells, only a small percentage of them, about three to 5 percent, may be the ones that expand tumor growth. If those few can be destroyed, then the tumor may be eliminated. Application of this knowledge may not reach clinical application for many years.[22]

No attempt has been made to cover data showing how prostate cancer might be prevented, although several factors may be involved: an active and healthy lifestyle, a moderate diet with more vegetables and fruit, reduced red meat consumption, lower saturated fat intake, and maintenance of a normal weight.

[22.] "Stem Cells That Kill," *Time*, April 24, 2006, 50–51.

Extensive research needs to be conducted before firm conclusions can be presented about prostate cancer prevention.

One example of how research findings must be examined carefully, including the source or sources of the data, comes from an article in which the writer stated, "Doctors have also cast doubt on the efficacy of prostate cancer screening tests and mammograms for women under the age of 50."[23] Well, that sentence gives one pause! Everyone knows what the writer meant, but a few word changes would have helped.

*   *   *

There are several major forms of prostate cancer treatment. Combinations of the following are often used, or one or more may be used in sequence when one method alone has not controlled the disease:

Surgery: complete removal of the gland via several surgical procedures, including laparoscopic surgery.

Radiation, often called external beam radiation of the gland.

Brachytherapy, which is the implantation of radiated seeds into the abdomen or directly into the prostate gland.

Hormone therapy to suppress testosterone.

Cryotherapy, which is freezing of the gland.

Heat therapy, which is heating the gland to a high temperature so that both cancerous and normal prostate cells are destroyed.

Chemotherapy, this medication may be used with one or more of the above treatments. Chemo is also increasingly used when cancer returns following previous treatment.

Watchful Surveillance. Previously called watchful waiting, this is the use of PSAs and DREs (prostate-specific exams and digital rectal exams) to determine whether, and how fast, a cancer may be growing. In effect, this is not a treatment, but an observation of tumor development.

---

23.   Western Wales Mail./Wales.icnetwork.co.uk/, August 24, 2005.

A discussion of these various therapies cannot be neatly described as in the above categories. A few of these can be described in isolation, but most are described in their combination with other forms of treatment.

Radiation

Radiation and hormone therapy are both included here, since they are so often combined as a treatment "package." A hormone to suppress or eliminate the major male hormone, testosterone, may be given before, during, and/or after a series of radiation treatments.

A five-year research project confirmed the major benefits of this common treatment that PC patients receive: radiation combined with hormone therapy. Almost one thousand six hundred men were studied in Boston, Massachusetts, and it was found that a "combined radiation therapy and androgen suppression therapy" is a more effective treatment for localized, early-stage prostate cancer compared to treatment using radiation therapy alone. Before this, the combination was used primarily on men with more advanced stages of cancer. This finding assures that there will be less treatment failures when both forms of treatment are used.[24]

While many studies examine short-term recovery from cancer, a greater emphasis is now being placed on long-term recovery. It is encouraging that combined treatments are increasingly being used and evaluated.

When radiation treatment is employed, the exact location of the prostate gland is extremely important. A new machine, given various names such as image-guided radiotherapy treatment, determines the precise location of the gland every second. The radiation treatment is then given within fifteen minutes of the assessment. The article notes that the gland may move as much as two to three millimeters or even five centimeters in a single day.[25] Movement of the gland depends on many factors, including a person's physical activities, amount of abdominal gas, volume of urine in the bladder and waste material in the bowel,

---

[24]   *http://www.sciencedaily.com/releases*, Dana-Farber Cancer Institute, Boston, MA, September 25, 2000. The Brigham and Women's Hospital shared in the project. Findings were published in the *Journal of the American Medical Association*, September 13, 2000. This treatment combination is the same one that I received.

[25]   www.varian.com, "Community Care Physicians of Latham, New York Deliver Ultra-Precise Image-Guided Radiotherapy Treatments for Prostate Cancer Patients," August 8, 2005.

and the movement of other internal organs. Fifteen of these machines are to be installed in locations throughout the world.[26]

An even more precise machine than the one above is under development but is yet to be tested in clinical practice. It holds promise of determining precisely where the gland is every second and then delivering the correct amount of radiation to the gland at the same time. This is in contrast to the device above that emits radiation fifteen minutes *after* the known location of the gland. The new machine's action, sometimes referred to as real-time imaging, would send almost no radiation to normal tissue.[27] This would probably eliminate some or all of the bowel and bladder problems that other men, including myself, have experienced with the current methods.

Still another machine, similar to those above, is called a TomoTherapy Hi-Art System. This 3.7-million-dollar device constantly changes the size, shape, and intensity of the radiation beam to conform to the exact same features of the tumor. One difference here is that the patient moves on a table into a radiation beam enclosed area, and the radiation is sent via hundreds of small beams in a circular area around the patient. With this new device, patients are in the enclosure for fifteen minutes.[28] This is the only combination treatment machine of its kind currently in the New York metropolitan area.[29] The very high cost of these machines shows good reason why they cannot be found in all communities.

A variation of the above machine is called a CyberKnife that "can reduce the number of radiation treatments from as many as forty over eight weeks to about five or less over one week." This equipment, which costs about six million dollars, is accurate within one millimeter and can move with a patient's breathing. Very few side effects have been reported. Radiation oncologist Robert Meier said that

---

26. In marked contrast to the new machines, X-rays were taken once a week to determine the location of my prostate gland. Consequently, some damage occurred to healthy tissue near the prostate.

27. http://seattlepi.nwsource.com/business/, June 1, 2005. A comparable Canadian-made device, costing over $300,000, was reported on July 14, 2005, and published on September 21, 2005, by GlobeandMail.com. The machine will be in both Vancouver Island and in Toronto, Canada.

28. In contrast I was on the radiation table in a large open area for about five minutes.

29. Journalnews.com, "Machine at Nyack Hospital Zeros in on Tumors," August 10, 2005.

the machine is quite flexible and can treat many tumors, other than prostate, that conventional machines cannot reach.[30]

The largest and most expensive—125 million dollars—radiation system will be installed at the M. D. Anderson Cancer Center in Houston, Texas, in 2006. Using superfast particles called protons, it has eight-foot-thick walls, and a pickup truck could drive through the area into which patients will be placed. It is the third one in the United States and is very controversial from both a treatment and cost perspective. Its power is immense; experts from the other two centers in New York and California state that this machine prevents a recurrence of prostate cancer. Studies of its advantages have been proved on only a small number of cancers. One-fourth of patients at the Houston center will be those with prostate cancer.[31]

A study by the American Society for Therapeutic Radiology and Oncology (ASTRO) found that a combination of three approaches: seed implants, external radiation, and hormone therapy is more effective than the two-treatment program. The lead author of the study, a radiation oncologist at a cancer center in Wheeling, West Virginia, stated that this combination helps "men with high-risk prostate cancer to live longer without the cancer returning." Nearly two hundred men with high-risk cancer were studied over eight years.[32]

A study from Australia and New Zealand shows how a different timing of therapies may improve treatment. In a four-year study of eight hundred patients, with a five-year follow-up analysis of eight hundred thousand data entries, it was learned that "for men with advanced cancer that had not spread beyond the prostate, six months hormone therapy *before* radiation therapy reduced death rates and the chance of the cancer spreading by a third, and cut the likelihood of it returning by 60 percent."[33] The study did not describe the

---

30. *www. The*Record.com, "Under the CyberKnife," Swedish Medical Center, Seattle, WA, May 19, 2006.

31. *www.HoustonChronicle.com,* "M. D. Anderson Private Venture Raises Questions," October 23, 2005.

32. Reported in the January 1, 2005, issue of the *International Journal of Radiation Oncology, Biology, Physics,* the official journal of ASTRO. *www.sciencedaily.com/ releases,* January 1, 2005.

33. *http://www.rednova.com/news,* May 22, 2005. The trial was conducted by David Lamb, oncologist from the Wellington School of Medicine in New Zealand. It was conducted in conjunction with the Trans-Tasman Cancer Group. In contrast to the above, my radiation began three months after the first hormone injection.

types of radiation equipment used nor what types of antiandrogen (hormones to suppress testosterone) medications were employed.

When a cancer spreads to the bones, moderate or severe pain will likely occur. Giving ten daily doses of thirty Gy (a measure of radiation power) has been found to minimize the pain. However, in a recent study of 898 patients, with either breast or prostate cancer, it was learned that a single dose of eight Gys gave as much pain relief as the thirty Gys. One-third of all patients treated in this matter no longer required narcotic medications. Two other results included: the retreatment rate was higher with the eight Gy, but the acute toxicity was less with eight Gy.[34]

Brachytherapy

Physicians are constantly searching for less invasive methods of treating all diseases. A new "high dose rate brachytherapy" gives patients in Portland, Maine, a choice of treatment closer to home. Doctors send a radioactive pellet along a tube smaller than two millimeters and place it in or near the cancer. It is used "most commonly (via a body orifice) to treat cancers of the lung, breast, prostate." This not only speeds up treatment for the patient, but there is no exposure of radiation to the therapists.[35] Surgical implantation of radioactive seeds are more typically placed in the abdomen via tiny incisions.

Hormone Therapy

Patients who receive hormone therapy are at increased risk for developing osteoporosis. Researchers from the Loyola University of Chicago Stritch School of Medicine noted that the disease is "characterized by brittle, easily fractured bones (and those features in turn) are associated with significant morbidity, mortality, and health care cost."[36] A study of 184 patients discovered that only about one of every

---

34. *www.cancerpage.com.* Study conducted at the Lutheran General Cancer Center, IL, June 8, 2005, "Shorter Duration Radiotherapy Suitable for Bone Mets Pain Relief," Reported in the June 2005 issue of the *National Cancer Institute,* 97:786–788. In a related editorial, two oncologists noted that this and two other related studies show that the single-dose therapy does control pain, "but it remains to be seen whether this approach will become the standard of care in the U.S."
35. *www.MaineToday.com,* "Potent Form of Radiation Therapy Available to Maine Cancer Patients," *Portland Press Herald,* June 22, 2005.
36. *www.50Connect.co.uk,* "Osteoporosis and the Prostate." October 10, 2005. January 2005 issue of *CANCER,* a peer review journal of the American Cancer Society.

seven patients received any osteoporosis management during hormone therapy. Researchers learned that very few oncologists address the problem, whereas "primary care physicians were the most aggressive at managing osteoporosis."[37] The authors encourage bone loss examinations on all patients receiving hormone therapy.

In an attempt to learn how quickly testosterone levels return to normal after hormone therapy, a provisional small study of fifteen male patients was conducted in 2005. The time to "initial testosterone detection ranged from six to twenty-two months." Normal testosterone levels were reached by six of the patients in a mean of seventeen and a half months.[38] Since testosterone provides energy and drive, this indicates the time it may take men to feel that they are "back to normal." Testosterone builds muscle mass and strength, contributes to sexual interest and ability, and helps to maintain bone density.

A treatment to decrease testosterone for patients whose cancer has spread beyond the prostate gland is the use of an implant named Viadur, which contains Lupron. This chemical is effective for one year; another implant can be inserted later. It is believed that the slow, smooth pace of the implant is preferable to the one-month or three-month injections. It is also less costly. The side effects include possible "male menopause—or even impotence." Some men find injections painful.[39] This report comes from the Chicago area, and both the American Cancer Society and the American Foundation for Urologic Disease were referenced.[40]

Heat Therapy

Another treatment method, that some compare to radiation, is called Ablatherm HIFU, or high intensity focused ultrasound, and is now available in

---

[37.] My family physician, Dr. Shah, had me take an exam immediately after completing radiation. I had a serious level of osteoporosis and was placed on medication to restore bone density and strength.

[38.] www.cancerpage.com, "Testosterone Stays Low After Stopping Prostate Cancer Hormone Therapy." Study source: British Journal of Urology, May 2005; 95:776–779. The therapy referred to here is called LH-RH or luteinizing hormone-releasing hormone analogues. It is one of several treatments included under the general term of hormone therapy.

[39.] Lupron is the hormone I received by injection. I had no discomfort with either the one-month or the three-month injections.

[40.] http://cbs2chicago.com/topstories, "Implant Slows Advanced Prostate Cancer," June 10, 2005.

Toronto, Canada. Originally developed in Europe, more than seven thousand patients have been successfully treated with this procedure. Patients are treated by a focused beam which rapidly raises the temperature in the prostate to eighty-five degrees Celsius. It essentially destroys prostate tissue. Only one treatment is given, lasting two to three hours, and the patient is released three hours later.[41] This treatment is not used extensively in the United States.

Watchful Surveillance

This passive method of treatment—it includes PSAs (protein-specific antigen blood test) and DREs (digital rectal exam)—is one of the most controversial. Two recent studies, described below, show the difference in research findings, thus making it difficult for patients and physicians to know whether to choose active intervention or to delay treatment until cancer appears to increase. Periodic ultrasound examination of the prostate gland, as well as a biopsy, may also be employed during the waiting period.

A nationwide study of survival data on 48,606 men between the ages of sixty-five to eighty was completed in early 2006 by researchers at the Fox Chase Medical Center in Philadelphia, Pennsylvania. The men were diagnosed with prostate cancer between 1991 and 1999. Dr. Yu-Ning Wong, a medical oncologist, found that all the men who were treated had "a distinct advantage over untreated patients." Median survival was ten years after diagnosis for those waiting, whereas those treated with surgery lived up to thirteen years longer. When Dr. Wong made adjustments to control "for age, race and marital status, treatment still trumped watchful waiting."[42] To support their findings, Dr. Wong referred to a randomized study that was consistent with the Fox Chase analysis. Seven hundred Scandinavians were studied for more than eight years, and the surgery group enjoyed a 44 percent higher survival rate. The latter study was published in the *New England Journal of Medicine* in 2005.

Dr. Gary Hughes, an oncologist and coauthor at the Fox Chase Center, explained that the "waiting game may actually be detrimental to men." He

---

41. *Financial News*, Maple Leaf HIFU Co., New York, NY, "Ablatherm® HIFU Prostate Cancer Treatment a Safe Alternative to Surgery or Radiotherapy," June 14, 2005. This is a substitute for surgery and has fewer complications than radical prostatectomy.

42. *www.consumerhealth@upi.com*, "Prostate Cancer Treatment Beats Waiting." Research by the Fox Chase Medical Center, Philadelphia, PA. Second reference: *www.Newsday.com*, "Prostate Cancer Therapy Trumps Wait," February 28, 2006.

added that men who are age seventy "could have an additional fourteen years of life—and so doctors can't think short term." In that same report, Dr. Gary Hughes, a prostate cancer researcher at the University of Toronto, advised that "many men with low-risk PC may not need treatment. A diagnosis of cancer does not always mean aggressive disease." Dr. Wong agreed that waiting is not passé, and "watchful waiting is still a legitimate option for some men." This study was presented at the 2006 Prostate Cancer Symposium in San Francisco.

Within a few days of the Fox Chase study, Johns Hopkins Hospital researchers came to the opposite conclusion. They stated that "men who had delayed surgery for more than two years did not increase their risk of noncurable prostate cancer compared with men who had surgery" three to four months after diagnosis.[43] The Hopkins report "compared 150 men with immediate surgery with thirty-eight men" who delayed surgery. The median age in both groups was sixty-one. This study was far more complex than the Fox Chase study in the number of variables examined, but it was miniscule when numbers of subjects are considered. The findings, explained by Dr. H. Ballentine Carter, are twofold: (1) Men diagnosed with early-stage PC should not believe their situation is urgent, and (2) Patients who delay surgery have the same risk of noncurable PC for at least two years after diagnosis. Another study mentioned in this report comes from a review of 767 men in Connecticut in 2005. It was concluded that there is "little harm in waiting or using hormone treatment instead of surgery." Thus, the issue of watchful surveillance remains unsettled.

The PSA remains controversial in terms of measuring the level of cancer and its accuracy in predicting the presence of disease. Researchers at Johns Hopkins University, Baltimore, Maryland, state that the test is "still the best method of predicting the likelihood of cancer recurrence after prostate surgery."[44] Stephen Freedland, MD, a clinical instructor in urology, explained that "PSA levels measured before prostate removal surgery were significantly associated with the risk of recurrent cancer after surgery. It certainly suggests that the PSA era is alive and well." He added that a single PSA "value is an extremely useful measure of a

---

43. *www.medpagetoday.com*, "Men with Localized Low-Grade Prostate Tumors Can Delay Surgery," March 1, 2006; Warlick et al. "Delayed Versus Immediate Surgical Intervention and Prostate Cancer Outcome," *Journal of the National Cancer Institute*, 98:355–7.

44. *www.mainemed.org.* Additional source: Johns Hopkins Medicine, news release, September 19, 2005 and September 23, 2005. It should be noted that this study is related primarily to use of the PSA following surgical removal of the prostate.

patient's risk of progression after surgery." In addition, the speed of increase, often called velocity, of the measure "over time is likely to be even more informative than a single value."

In the fall of 2004, the Mayo Clinic reported on an antidepressant, named paroxetine, that has been used for women to manage hot flashes. It has not yet been studied in men. In a very small study, researchers found male hot flashes reduced from over six a day to less than three. The severity of flashes, based on a numerical score, decreased in the same time from a score of 10.6 to 3 per day. They noted that hot flashes in males undergoing "androgen ablation therapy, also known as hormonal deprivation therapy" are well known but treatment of the flashes have not been studied.[45] This project is one that should be considered with caution, since control groups were not used and the number of patients was so small. There was no examination of side effects of the medication, and long-term clinical study would be required to determine its true benefits. It nevertheless offers hope for a resolution of a problem which seems to plague most men who undergo hormone therapy.

The following material presents very short descriptions of other findings, without referencing all the details. Studies presented in 2005 at a national professional meeting[46] include

1. Analyses of patients with high-grade PC following three approaches—watchful waiting, prostatectomy, and radiation—concluded that surgical removal of the gland has a higher survival advantage.[47]

2. When controlling for PC that has not spread, African American men are more likely to develop PC than Caucasian men. However, socioeconomic factors such as insurance and income may account for some racial disparity outcomes.

3. Men who have a family history of cancer and who also have a family history of PC (such as a brother or father) are more likely to have

---

45. *www.ScienceDaily.com*, May 23, 2005. Additional source: *Mayo Clinic Proceedings*, a peer review publication, Rochester, MN, October 19, 2004.

46. *www.myDNA.com*, News Center, "Variables and Options for Prostate Cancer," 100th Annual Meeting of the American Urological Association, May 2005.

47. This conclusion is interesting in that more men are treated currently with radiation.

less severe disease complications at the time of a prostatectomy, when compared to patients with no family history. They also have higher levels of disease-free survival. This may not appear logical, but it is likely that men with a known family history seek treatment earlier than they otherwise would.

4. In a study to assess the importance of age at time of treatment, it was found that age is not a factor in outcomes after surgical removal of the gland. It was learned that the severity of the cancer and the grade are worse in older populations, and those two characteristics play a major role in all postoperative success.

Probably one of the most beneficial advances in many fields of medicine will come from personalized medicine that will include analyses of the unique cell composition in each person. Scientists have discovered that "people's genes show small variations in their nucleotide (DNA base) content." Therefore, genetic testing for predicting a person's response to drugs is now possible. The name of this new scientific approach is pharmacogenomics. It examines the "inherited variations in genes that dictate drug response and explores the ways those variations can be used to predict whether a patient will have a good response to a drug, a bad response to a drug, or no response at all."[48] For example, "once a patient is diagnosed with prostate, colon . . . cancer, etc., a secondary diagnostic test will be employed to discover what the individual's response to a particular treatment will be."[49]

This may be the ultimate form of treatment, but it may be one or two decades before it is readily available everywhere and for all patients. The real promise of this approach is that patients will no longer receive one-size-fits-all procedures or medications but ones that are tailored to each person's unique constitution and metabolism. Furthermore, follow-up amelioration of recognized and anticipated problems resulting from the treatment will be in place.

A beginning approach to gene utilization is taking place in a Vermont study. A vaccine for control of cancer is described as being on the near horizon; the treatment is composed of "genetically modified prostate cancer cells that are

---

[48]. *www.ncbi.nLm.N.H.Gov/About/primer/pharm.* This is the webpage of the National Center for Biotechnology Information.

[49]. *www.pharmaline.com*, MedAd News, July 25, 2005, 14th Annual Report on the Top Biotechnology Companies, Newtown, PA.

injected into the skin to provoke a response by the body's immune system." Those cells then locate and destroy active cancer cells. Early trials seemed promising, and about six hundred men are currently enrolled in a nationwide trial.[50] In a separate study by federal scientists at the National Cancer Institute, the vaccine was combined with hormone treatment. Control over cancer was maintained almost twice as long as treatment without the vaccine. Researchers noted that the vaccine is not intended to prevent cancer from occurring but is designed to stop recurrence of the disease.[51] Researchers stated that larger studies are needed to confirm the effectiveness of this approach.

A second report by Dr. Eric Small, University of California, San Francisco, on this same vaccine, noted that it "prolongs life yet avoids the side effects of other therapeutic approaches."[52] Dr. Small maintains that "this approach will be attractive to both patients and physicians."

A further implementation of genetic analysis is expected to emerge from an interorganizational study at the University of California, Irvine.[53] The goal is to develop a "gene signature" of PC for recently diagnosed patients based on a "tumor biopsy or blood examination. This signature will let patients know if they have an aggressive form of cancer—allowing them to better understand their disease and to make crucial decisions for appropriate early stage treatment." In short, this will be a genetic method for *predicting the outcome of prostate cancer at the time of diagnosis*. This important project may help to answer concerns that many cancer specialists have about the accuracy and usefulness of the PSA test. This is a five-year 9.5-million-dollar grant from the National Cancer Institute. Dr. Dan Mercola, the lead investigator, stated that this will meet a critical unmet need in PC treatment: "Up to 30 percent of men with PC do not need radical treatments like radiation or surgery, and this test will allow us to determine" who they are.

---

50. *www.rutlandherald.com*, September 25, 2005. The Southwestern Vermont Medical Center, Bennington, Vermont, seeks men willing to participate in the study.

51. *www.rednova.com/news/display*. The article also referenced the Prostate Cancer Foundation and the Laboratory of Tumor Immunology and Biology at the National Cancer Institute, Bethesda, Maryland. Reported in the August 2005 *Journal of Urology*.

52. *www.sciencedaily.com*, "Prostate Cancer Vaccine Is First to Increase Survival," March 2, 2005.

53. *www.medicalnewstoday.com*, "UCI Receives Major Grant to Develop 'Gene Signature' for Prostate Cancer Prognosis," February 13, 2005.

*   *   *

These varied studies can seem very confusing since they are so diverse in size, scope, number, and characteristics of patients, type of treatment or treatments, as well as the recognized commitments or convictions of some cancer specialists to a certain approach.

In truth, the above studies and projects show positive, encouraging developments and advancements in cancer care. Research is ongoing and increasingly expansive. A national meeting on PC was called in the spring of 2005 by prominent leaders and specialists from Johns Hopkins University, the American Cancer Society, the Dana-Farber Cancer Institute in Boston, the University of California, and the U.S. National Cancer Institute.[54] Over one thousand persons attended. Leaders expressed concern that PC knowledge and treatment programs are at least twenty years behind those in breast cancer, and "prostate cancer gets a fraction of what is spent on breast cancer research, and virtually nothing is known about what causes it." Members hoped to acquire more funding and to boost the visibility of PC, just as breast cancer is so well known and supported in the United States. Leaders compared this current meeting to one held twenty-seven years ago on breast cancer.

That year, 1978, was the start of annual meetings on breast cancer, the initiation of breast cancer public knowledge, and the funding of substantial research and treatment. Members in the 2005 PC conference anticipated that the same changes and breakthroughs would occur following this meeting.

While the prostate cancer field does not have all that is needed, there is certainly strong evidence of great vigor and commitment to the study, treatment, and control of prostate cancer. Those efforts will inevitably expand to the reduction and possible prevention of prostate cancer.

[54.]   *Boston Sunday Globe*, Boston, MA, March 27, 2005, 21.

INDEX

E

ED. *See* erectile dysfunction
effects of hormone therapy
    changes in cognition and mood 39
    decreased libido 38
    delayed toxicity 39
    enlargement of male breast tissue 39
    hot flashes 39, 50, 51, 57, 71, 77, 80,
        89, 131
    impotence 38
    metabolic alterations 39
    nausea 39
    osteopenia 39
    osteoporosis 39, 149
    peripheral swelling 39
    testicular atrophy 39
    tiredness and low energy 39
    transient bone pain 39
    vomiting 39
effects of radiation
    diarrhea 38
    hair loss 38
    uncomfortable urination 38
erectile dysfunction 27
external beam radiation 145
external beam radiotherapy 37
external radiation 148

F

Flomax 87
Fox Chase analysis 151
Fox Chase Medical Center 151
Freedland, Stephen 152

G

garden-variety cancer 58
general physical exam 17
gene signature 155

genitourinary system 16
Gleason score 24
Gy 149

H

Harrison, Rex 101
HIFU. *See* high intensity focused
    ultrasound
high-techtable 41
high intensity focused ultrasound 150
hot flashes 45, 50, 51, 52, 57, 71, 73, 77,
    78, 80, 89, 90, 95, 112, 131, 133,
    134, 136
Hughes, Gary 151
hypertrophic disease 17

I

image-guided radiotherapy treatment
    146
In Celebration of the Cancer Center 105
internal radiation 37
irritable mood 81, 82

J

Johns Hopkins Hospital 152
Johns Hopkins University 152, 156
Journal of the American Medical Association
    38

K

Kauffman, Richard A. 109
Kenyon, Jane 107, 108, 109

L

leuprolide suspension 80
linear accelerator 42, 44